Painless Childbirth

AN EMPOWERING JOURNEY THROUGH PREGNANCY AND BIRTH

Giuditta Tornetta

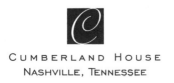

CUMBERLAND HOUSE
NASHVILLE, TENNESSEE

PAINLESS CHILDBIRTH
PUBLISHED BY CUMBERLAND HOUSE PUBLISHING
431 Harding Industrial Drive
Nashville, Tennessee 37211

Library of Congress Cataloging-in-Publication Data
Tornetta, Giuditta, 1956–
  Painless childbirth : an empowering journey through pregnancy and birth / Giuditta Tornetta.
       p. cm.
   ISBN-13: 978-1-58182-640-1 (pbk. : alk. paper)
   ISBN-10: 1-58182-640-0 (pbk. : alk. paper)
   1. Natural childbirth. I. Title.

   RG661.T67 2008
   618.4'5—dc22

                                                        2008002670

Printed in the United States of America
1 2 3 4 5 6 7—14 13 12 11 10 09 08

To my children Azzurro and Natascia:
my best teachers and the loves of my life

CONTENTS

FOREWORD

This is a wonderful book. Giuditta Tornetta has combined body, mind, and spirit in a manner that touches at the very heart of what it means to bring another human being into the world. She recognizes how beliefs, emotions, and behaviors can hinder or enhance a woman's experience of birth. Every woman expecting a baby should read this book. Giuditta takes you on a journey to explore your fears and any barriers between you and the birth that is possible for you and your baby. She helps you with healing those fears. Additionally, maternity caregivers, be they doctors, midwives, or nurses, who meet the woman as she faces this immense transformative event will gain more understanding of their power to help or hurt the woman in this vulnerable state of releasing her baby into the world.

Support people, partners, and doulas will also benefit by having a greater depth of knowledge of the potential of their roles and how to provide the appropriate support as they travel on the journey of birth with the woman.

The personal stories are both instructive and inspirational. Stories are an important way to engage the mind, body, senses, and emotions and provide learning at a deeper level where there is a sensory and physiological identification. Women will gain more confidence to trust in their body's natural wisdom.

PHYLLIS KLAUS, MFT, CSW

PERINATAL THERAPIST, RESEARCHER, AUTHOR:

YOUR AMAZING NEWBORN, BONDING,

THE DOULA BOOK, WHEN SURVIVORS GIVE BIRTH

PREFACE

Millions of women all over the world have experienced a natural and painless childbirth. If you would like to join this growing number, this is the right book for you.

When I talk about a painless childbirth, I don't mean you will not feel anything. You'll experience each wave as surges of incredible energy. You'll innately know how labor comes one minute at a time, and when you focus on managing that one minute, you'll be able to conquer it. Childbirth is a natural event with a known positive outcome. While a contraction is indeed intense, it lasts only one minute and then you get a break—guaranteed. When you learn to manage these contractions one minute at a time, you learn that labor is very different from what you have experienced as pain in your life.

Pain is usually what we feel when something goes wrong. It is often associated with an unknown outcome: When we break a leg, we feel pain and there is no reprieve unless we resort to painkillers. We wonder how long it will take before we can again walk normally. How long or if we will be able to go back to our regular activities.

By contrast, in birth, once the baby comes out, the sensations of labor go away and you have a happy, amazing, loving baby snuggling in your arms. Painlessness is a state of well-being that encompasses body, mind, and spirit.

When I was pregnant with my son, I experienced my soul slowly recognizing its higher potentiality as this child was forming inside my womb. It was exciting to feel the power of creation within me. I learned to relate to him as I would relate to an angel. If I lived my life asking myself, "What are my actions, beliefs, thoughts, and attitudes teaching my child right now?" I would embark on a journey that would not only birth a better human being, but birth a new self.

Eastern religions speak of the Divine not as an entity outside of us, but as something we are a part of, something that is closer than our hands and feet, nearer than our breath. This abstract concept became very real as I felt my baby growing in my belly, and I felt his touch and movements. Being a creator of a human life awakened in me the awareness that my body was a vessel for the miracle of creation and the nine months of gestation a unique opportunity to learn the secret of conscious living.

This spiritual awakening was instrumental in my ability to experience a painless childbirth. When I speak of spiritual awakening and close contact with my Higher Power, I am referring to a Higher Love that encompasses all. Sometimes I call it God, or Higher Power, or Mother Nature. I encourage you to find your personal connection with a power greater than yourself. Being spiritually enlightened and leading a conscious life can be done as a Christian, Jew, Muslim, Hindu, Buddhist, and even an agnostic. What you call it, how you refer to it, how you pray to it does not matter. What matters is that you feel the power of creation within you and become one with this power. Seek your own relationship with the Divine—you don't need any intermediary.

I have designed this book to support you as you delve into the excitement and exhilaration of pregnancy and birth. It is my intention to guide you through your fears and occasional feelings of unworthiness, as well as your moments of elation and anticipation as we celebrate, laugh, cry, and smile together. Don't be concerned if you don't entirely understand each concept, each step or basic human right. This work is intuitive and sometimes the intellect stands in the way of our deep understanding. Be patient with yourself. Some stories will immediately ring true, while others might seem far off from your experience. Yet they all offer tools you can use to your advantage. Give yourself the time to contemplate, and meditate on some of the concepts. Some months will be easier than others; be gentle with yourself and mother yourself as you mother your child.

Each month starts and ends with an affirmation, or hypnotic suggestion, designed to prepare you for a painless childbirth experience. I encourage you to read them once, then close your eyes and let them sink in. They are designed to speak directly to your Higher Self. There is no perfect way to navigate this book, nor a right way to birth your baby. There is only *your* way and Nature's way and they are one and the same.

This book was made possible by hundreds of couples who allowed me the honor of witnessing the birth of their children. All the stories in this book are true, but nearly all names have been changed to respect my clients' anonymity.

One of the universal laws states: if one person can do it, it can be done by others. I say to you: I have experienced a painless childbirth, now so can you.

ACKNOWLEDGMENTS

The idea for this book was born at the same time as my daughter Natascia; her birth had been completely painless and I knew I wanted to share my experience with other women. Twenty-three years later, my dream has come true. I want to thank first and foremost both of my children, Azzurro and Natascia; without their inspiration I could not have written this book. In the past few months leading up to the delivery of the manuscript, they have both been so supportive, editing my words and even suggesting many important changes. Azzurro is responsible for the affirmation preceding every chapter. Natascia has kept me conscious and present for every page. I am so grateful to my first editor, Linda Arvanites, who believed in my project even when I got discouraged, and my agent, Natasha Kern, who fell in love with the book right away. This book would not have been possible without the support of all of my clients. I have learned so much from them and feel honored to have been part of the miracle they've experienced in pregnancy and childbirth.

I would like to acknowledge the following individuals and associations who either directly or indirectly enlightened me in so many ways: Phyllis Klaus; Dr. Jay Gordon;

Dr. Harvey Karp; Dr. Christiane Northrup; Kimber Shining Star; Elisabeth Day, my final editor; the Doulas Association of Southern California; Doulas of West Los Angeles; Diana Payne; my spiritual center, Agape; Reverend Dr. Michael Beckwith; and all the teachers, speakers, and people who have inspired me and comforted me in the long years of preparation for this book. A special thanks to my publisher Ron Pitkin, who understood the importance of this book's title; Annette, who helped me look not only at the writing but at its visual presentation. Finally, I would like to acknowledge my mother, Anna Tornetta, and my father, Ennio Tornetta, for bringing me into this world; and last but not least I am grateful to the nuns that raised me; without them I could not have embraced God the way I did.

Painless Childbirth

INTRODUCTION

THE PATH IS REVEALED

I had started writing a book about my painless birthing experience after my daughter's birth, but the job of raising my children and financially providing for them took over my life. I put the book into hibernation until one day my life took a dramatic turn. It all began after I was let go from my latest job and was at a loss as to what to do next. One of my saving graces in life has been taking a morning walk and having a conversation with God. I asked, "What do you want me to do next? I am willing to work hard, so why am I not getting a job? How can I provide for my children?" What I heard was, "Be patient and listen. Follow whatever suggestion you hear next."

God talks to us through people, places, and things. So, when an acquaintance suggested I look into getting a certificate in Lactation Education at UCLA, I did it without asking any questions. At that point in my life I had been earning a solid six-figure salary and I was fully aware that lactation education was more a vocation than a profession. But I have learned never to question my Higher Power, and I soon found out where the magic was. In that class, I met a doula[1] who spoke of her job as an amazing mission of love, helping women bring their children naturally into this world without the use of drugs or medical intervention. I realized this was the answer to my lifelong desire to share my painless experience with other women.

As I decided to embrace that profession wholeheartedly, my daughter found my first client—the universe's response was immediate. A few weeks before this client's due date, I drove all the way to San Francisco and attended a certification course to become a birth doula. As a rite of passage, that first birth was one of the most challenging to date: a thirty-nine hour labor that culminated in a Cesarean birth—a decision made more by an annoyed doctor than due to a medical reason. With my encouragement, my teenage client had been surrounded by her dearest friend, and the doctor was outspoken in his annoyance of the crowd helping the laboring woman. Shaken by witnessing this woman's ordeal and outright abuse by the medical institution, I looked to the heavens and asked, "Why are you doing this to me?" "It's not about you," was the response. Understanding that helped me take my ego out of the equation.

I began to find clients without much effort. Doula mentors appeared, and people gave me books and videos about alternative ways of birthing. Workshops about how to build your own business, postpartum care, childbirth education, and neonatal CPR came my way. Friends were cheering me on. It seemed that the universe was conspiring for my success. I created a Web site and began writing articles about alternative ways to birth. The law of attraction was in full force.

My book was still on my mind, but I needed more guidance for its structure. Once again I asked for direction during my meditation practice.

THE CHAKRAS

In my years of practicing yoga, I have learned about the chakras and their influence on our physical and spiritual well-being. A chakra is a center of activity that receives, assimilates, and expresses life-force energy. The word *chakra* literally translates as "wheel" or "disk" and refers to a spinning sphere of bioenergetics activity emanating from various centers in the human body. These bioenergetics centers are aligned with the spinal column, from the base of the spine to the top of the head. Most Eastern healers, and now quite a few Western ones, propose that there is a correlation between the seven chakras of the human body and the spiritual and physical well-being of a person. It is said that when we become conscious of the blockages within each center, and we are willing to do the emotional and spiritual work to clear those blockages, we can obtain deep and incredible healing of body and mind. In my search for a structure to suggest a healing path to pregnant women, I felt I was onto something with the chakras, but still needed more clarity, so I went boogie-boarding.

I love boogie-boarding and the three specific rituals that go with it. First, you swim out to the place where you'll wait for the wave. This can be challenging, because at times the waves seem to oppose your desire to get to where you want to go. When they were really strong and slapped me back to shore, my mind would mock me: "Get out of the water, old lady! Behave your own age!" Despite that annoying voice in my head, I would wrestle my way through and fight for my right to boogie-board, regardless of anyone's judgment, including my own.

The second ritual is the meditative calm all surfers experience while waiting for the wave. There is little dialogue between surfers out there. It is a personal moment, a great moment cuddled in the arms of the ocean. There I have had my best conversations with Father/Mother/God. That's where I embraced my right to feel one with the beautiful ocean, with the universe, and with the Divine.

Finally, I see her, my wave, the one I decide to ride all the way to shore. I size it up and wonder if it is sizing me up. All thoughts are gone, and only my innate trust that I can surf it remains. I know the ritual: I turn, I swim to match its speed, and then I let it take me as I experience exhilaration, pure freedom, and trust in my Divine right to act and have the "ride of my life."

And there it was: I had just fulfilled three basic human rights—the right to act, the right to want, and the right to feel. What I had just experienced allowed me to see a parallel between the basic rights attached to the chakras and the steps a woman must take to be a conscious creator of her baby and experience a painless childbirth. Once at home, I looked at the phases of the growing fetus in the womb and I discovered that there was a miraculous parallel between the baby's development and the lessons encased in each chakra. If we are all made up of energy and if we can manipulate our energy through emotional and spiritual states, then by learning the lessons in our seven energy centers (the chakras), we can contribute to imbuing the baby's every fiber with a specific healing energy.

THE NINE CHAKRAS AND THE NINE MONTHS OF PREGNANCY

Quantum physics suggest that energetic fields are the very basic substance of the universe. The concept of an "energetic field" arose in Western science when electrons were observed to repel other electrons but attract protons according to their needs. These needs spring forth from the information stored in the protons.

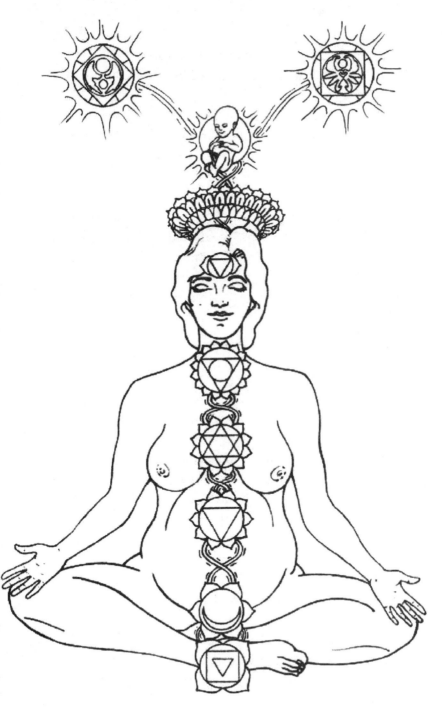

THE NINE CHAKRAS

Knowing that our body is an electromagnetic field that responds to stimuli, we can deduce that on a larger scale we also attract or repel that which we need based on the information that is stored within us. Let's look at how we gather, categorize, store, and distribute information. First, information is processed with our five senses. The data is then received by our mind, which categorizes and labels it using acquired knowledge and our deductive abilities. Then, it is passed through our emotions, which are tied to our memories. The emotions create a biochemistry that runs through our bloodstream and informs our entire body. For example, when we look at a computer we first see its physical aspects and we take in information about its colors, shapes, width, height, depth, luminosity, and other physical characteristics. Passing this visual information through our mind, knowledge, and experience, we further know that this object can be used to communicate, write, research information, and watch images. The next filter is an emotional one. If we are familiar with the object, we feel good about it and we sense it as a simple tool that makes our modern living easier. If we feel intimidated by this object, we project a negative feeling toward it because it creates frustration, and we categorize it as bad or a calamity of progress. If we were to constantly receive bad news from this object, we'd fear it as something that only brings doom and bad tidings. Our emotions create a relation-

THE MORE WE UNDERSTAND ABOUT THE FUTURE CONSEQUENCES OF WHAT WE ARE DOING, AND THE INTENT THAT GOES WITH THE ACTION, THE MORE SUCCESSFUL WE WILL BE IN CARING FOR OUR CHILDREN WITH OUR OWN PURPOSES AND GOALS OF PARENTING IN MIND. PARENTS NEED TO DECIDE TOGETHER WHAT THEY BELIEVE TO BE A HEALTHY HUMAN BEING.

DOTTY COPLEN, *PARENTING FOR A HEALTHY FUTURE*

ship with the object tied to our memory. The same goes with everything we observe. At times this process is fast and unconscious and our reactions come from a memory that is deeply imbedded in our unconscious. Thus, our relationship with all that crosses our path is filtered through our acquired knowledge stored in our memory, and our relationship toward it depends on experience.

Through the study of perinatal and prenatal psychology we know that the embryo begins learning and accumulating memory from the very beginning of its life in utero. Therefore, our personal choices and actions when pregnant have significant impact upon the forming of the baby, his future, his coping mechanisms, his ability to grow and learn, and his relationship with all that surrounds him. We can conclude then that some of our reactions are tied to a memory that might not even be ours, but one that belonged to our mothers.

When we consider our body as an electromagnetic field that contains seven energy centers, or chakras, we can see how during pregnancy all chakras are activated in the creation of another human being. Furthermore, the addition of our baby's chakras not only changes our biochemistry, but the process of creation becomes a dance of information given and received from one body, mind, and soul to the other.

As I carefully watched hundreds of mommies-to-be, I saw that their chakras were emanating incredible energy, amplified by the baby's own chakras inside the belly. As I focused further, I saw that there were not just seven chakras, but nine: two chakras hovered over the woman's shoulders, like guardian angels accompanying her on her journey from pregnancy to birth. When I meditated on the nature of these other two chakras, I recognized that the additional two above the seventh chakra have a Divine quality. In essence, God provides celestial assistants to each woman when she embodies the Divine quality of being a creator. I began envisioning these two chakras as a funnel, an inverted triangle, which is also the most ancient symbol of the feminine, through which the Divine would enter directly and become incarnate.

Research has shown that the emotional stability in each of the parents at the time of conception and pregnancy is most important for healthiest development of the embryo and placenta.[2] As the baby grows in the womb, it is the parent's responsibility and the one chance in a lifetime to grow, learn, and change as the baby does.

Let's look at the correlation between the chakras and the baby's growth. Each month, the baby's phases of development in utero recall specific characteristics of each chakra. As the nine chakras are associated with a set of desires and lessons that go from primordial to Divine, the baby's growth goes from basic survival to oneness with the Divine. When you look at Table 1 and follow it horizontally, you can see this correlation.

After nearly twenty years of personal research, I began to synthesize this revelation to create specific tools that would help women navigate through their pregnancy. Using the chakras as the starting point, we can heal ourselves and teach our children the tools for self-confidence, serenity, and self-healing. This nine-step guide is the road map I used to have a painless, conscious, and sacred birth. Each month relates to one of the nine basic human rights, bringing together several modalities, exercises, inspirational stories, and personal experiences to advance in the quest for conscious creation.

Just as if I were your doula, this book is meant to be an intimate conversation between the two of us. I'll be answering some of your questions and relating stories to nurture your spiritual growth. I encourage you to take charge of your pregnancy and birthing experience. Many spiritual teachers, avatars, and even modern quantum physicists

TABLE 1

Chakras	Placement	Quality/ Lesson	Basic Human Right	Gestational Month	Baby Growth In Utero
First	Base of the spine	Survival	To have and to be here	0 to 4 weeks	Beating heart and yolk sac—life and sustenance
Second	Above the belly button	Emotions toward the "other"	To feel and to want	4 to 8 weeks	Baby's arms and fingers are formed to touch the "other"
Third	Solar plexus	Personal power	To act	8 to 12 weeks	Baby is displaying the actions of interest and of protest as a result of experiences
Fourth	Heart	Love	To love and be loved	12 to 16 weeks	Baby's sexuality is defined as boy or girl
Fifth	Throat	Sound	To speak and hear the truth	16 to 20 weeks	Baby kicks mom's belly and begins tangible communication
Sixth	Third eye	Sight and insight	To see and know the truth	20 to 24 weeks	Baby can see and reacts to light
Seventh	Crown of the head	Consciousness	To live consciously	24 to 28 weeks	Baby's brain is fully functioning
Eighth	Two feet above left shoulder	Divine	To Divine powers	28 to 32 weeks	Baby dreams metaphysical visions
Ninth	Two feet above right shoulder	Incarnation	To be one with the Divine	32 to 36 weeks	Baby is ready to be the creator of her own reality

teach us that we cannot know, love, or care for another unless we know, love, and care for ourselves. On an airplane, parents are instructed that in case of an emergency they should place the oxygen mask on themselves before helping their child. I encourage you to embark on a journey of self-discovery before caring for a new child. Each chapter reveals the next step, the ensuing connection, and where to find the spiritual common denominator. As we heal ourselves, we can heal the world.

CONCEPTION

SCIENTIFIC STUDIES SUPPORT SPIRITUAL ENLIGHTENMENT

Recently, I was attending a presentation entitled "Early Childhood Influences on a Woman's Later Childbearing" by my mentor and dear friend, Penny Simkin.[3] She explained the following:

> Events of pregnancy and birth have a profound and lasting impact on the person as she grows to adulthood. Research illustrates that often adults who had a traumatic birthing experience will experience similar complications once they give birth. Studies have also shown that "resilient women," those who did not repeat their own negative birthing experience, had one or more of the following four attributes in common:
>
> 1. They had a significant adult figure in their lives who made them feel "safe" during childhood.
> 2. They had been raised in a non-gender typified family where "girls are equal to boys."
> 3. They had significant episodes of success in activities that ranged from sport to business and/or artistic expression.
> 4. They exhibited a strong faith in the Divine.[4]

Thanks to the fourth attribute, I realized that I am one of those resilient women. I was able to create the ideal environment, both physically and spiritually, to define my own birthing experience and greatly differentiate it from the one my mother had.

MY STORY

Both of my children were born at home, with the help of a midwife. From the very moment I conceived my son, the journey was one of wondrous discovery and self-realization. When it came time to deliver him into this world, the labor was surprisingly intense. He was in a posterior presentation,[5] which is known to be much more challenging than the anterior presentation. Even though my labor with him was intense, I settled into a rhythm that helped me manage each contraction as unique expressions of his coming into this world. This amazing first experience prepared me for my daughter's birth, two years later. Knowing what to expect and trusting that my body was created for this task, I was able to completely surrender to the miracle unfolding and obtain a painless childbirth. In fact, after preparing myself throughout the nine months of pregnancy, I can confidently say that I experienced true joy in birthing.

The knowledge I had acquired during the pregnancy and delivery of my son helped me become more conscious and in charge of my body and mind. Thus when my daughter was ready to be born I approached the event with a true sense of oneness with the divine force within me. When my labor started, and as the contractions intensified, I got on my knees and began to chant the sound "Ah." I had not heard it before; it came out of my lips on its own. It helped me breathe at regular intervals. My body would go limp as I chanted, "Ahhhhh, ahhhh." I tuned in and listened to the guidance that had shown up when my water had broken that morning and the contractions had begun. These contractions were strong and powerful, yet I was directed not to think of them as pain, but rather as magical and extraordinary feelings. The guidance I had sought daily to improve my conscious contact with the divine was present and in charge. In retrospect I recognized that chanting and trusting in the divine process kept me in the moment—one minute at a time, one contraction at a time. The results were amazing—almost unbelievable. *A painless childbirth.*

As women we have a unique quality–our innate ability to give birth to our children naturally, painlessly, and even effortlessly. I wanted to share my journey with other women and tell them that when we consider pregnancy, birth, and parenting as a spiritual practice we can obtain what some think impossible—a painless childbirth. I am no spiritual leader or guru, so when it came to writing about a spiritual practice I did not feel prepared. After all, as with many people, my relationship with the Divine, or the G word, was one mixed with hurtful memories, unanswered questions, and skepticism. I first had to understand the origins of my faith.

MY FIRST EXPERIENCE WITH THE DIVINE

When I was five years old, my parents were determined to give me the best schooling available, so they chose L'Institute Du Sacre Coeur De Jésus (the Institute of the Sacred Heart of Jesus), a very exclusive Catholic school run by French nuns. The schedule was Monday through Saturday, 9:00 a.m. to 4:30 p.m. In addition to the regular curriculum, I was to study French and catechism.

The institute was a beautiful building on the hills of Turin, Italy, sculpting the backdrop of the Gran Paradiso Mountain. The gardens were an immense playground with blossoming cherry trees in the spring, primrose flowers announcing the first sun of the year, ponds with goldfish, and innumerable steps, bridges, creeks, and evergreen giants. Nature's beauty was everywhere. The building was a sixteenth century convent that smelled of musk and echoed with children's laughter. Made of marble and stone, the school was four stories high. A theater and offices were located on the ground floor, preschool and elementary on the second floor, middle school on the third, and high school on the forbidden fourth floor. Each floor could be conquered and explored only once you reached the appropriate grade. If anyone was found on "higher ground," there were consequences to be paid.

One day sitting in my classroom in kindergarten surrounded by classmates, I asked the nun to be excused for a bathroom break. I left the classroom and inched my way toward the great staircase leading up to the forbidden territory. It was nearly dark as the winter sun set earlier in the day. By four o'clock, there were plenty of shadowy dark places looming and beckoning. The challenge I had pledged with my classmates was to run as fast as possible up the stairs and discover the mysteries of the high school floor. Once at the top, I would be alone and unsupervised. I looked down the staircase, first making sure no one was coming up from the first floor, quickly glanced at my floor, and then without hesitation I ran the two flights of stairs up to the fourth floor. I must have held my breath the entire way, for once there, I nearly fainted. The corridor was dark and silent because the high school session ended at one in the afternoon. Walking slowly, I peeked into a few rooms to see what forbidden treasures they held, but they all seemed to look pretty much the same as the two floors below.

Suddenly I heard a noise and ran into the bathroom.

Their bathroom was very similar to ours, but the toilets were higher and they had a small closet next to the sink. It was a white metal closet, and initially I did not pay much attention to it. I walked toward the toilet, pulled my knickers down, and sat on the bowl trying to figure out what I was going to tell my friends. They were all waiting to find out what I had found. As I contemplated which story to tell I looked again at that closet. That was the only major difference I had noticed between the floors, at least in the bathroom. I reasoned that the secret must have been contained inside that otherwise common piece of furniture. I got up, flushed the toilet, and approached the metal doors. I reached for the shiny flat knob and opened it slowly. Inside I found extra toilet paper, one extra towel roll, and a pink box. I held the box in my hands. First I smelled it and then slowly I opened it and saw what I thought was a small pillow made of gauze and of cotton. I examined this strange new object, trying to assess its purpose and, most importantly, its forbidden use. I heard the creaking of the bathroom door and cringed. One of the assistant nuns had heard the toilet flushing and had run upstairs. Panting, she towered over me in her grey habit, with her thick black-rimmed glasses and a shadow of mustache budding on her upper lip.

"Tornetta, what are you doing?" she rasped.

"Mmm, I, I . . . I had to pee?"

"Don't lie to me," she bellowed. "Lying is a mortal sin! You deserve to be punished!"

She took me by the hand and we flew down two flights of stairs to my classroom, the strange object still in my other hand. She flung me into the corner for time-out and I was instructed to put my hands into prayer position. She ordered me not to move, and I found myself holding the evidence between my palms. She rounded the corner as a dark tornado, her black veil flapping in her self-generating storm. In her hands she was holding a small dark bottle. She rubbed some of the oily contents of the bottle on my conjoined hands and bound them together using some gauze.

"If you move, your hands will be deformed," she whispered in my ears.

The ointment smelled rancid, even wicked. Looking down at my hands with terror and nauseated by the unpleasant smell, I closed my eyes and began praying deeply to baby Jesus.

"Dear baby Jesus," I whispered, careful not to be overheard, "please forgive me. I'll never be bad again."

I was not sure what deformed meant, but I knew it had to be bad. If I went home with my hands somehow changed, my dad would kill me. As a five-year-old child I experienced time passing by slowly and inexorably. The loud noises of my rambunctious classmates, who wanted to know what I was holding in my hands, disturbed my concentration. If I so much as turned my head I was in sure danger of moving my hands. No one but the nun and I knew what could befall me.

To distract myself I fantasized that I was the statue of the Virgin Mary, between plaster clouds and pallid angels, standing triumphantly in the corner of the chapel. I smiled, I relaxed, I got bored, I nodded off, I moved! My entire body cringed in fear. I pleaded once more, "Baby Jesus, forgive me."

Had my fate been decided? I asked myself, but nothing seemed to happen, and as I looked down, my hands seemed the same. Maybe deformed meant that they would change color, I wondered. All I could see were the tips of my fingers, but they were just as pink as before. Discreetly, yet defiantly, I shook my hands. Bored, I began toying with fate and shook them vigorously. Would Jesus side with me—or with the wicked nun?

After what seemed like days, the head Sister approached from behind, turned me gently around, and removed the gauze. Ironically, the object I was still holding in my hands I later discovered represented my entrance into womanhood. Relived, I saw that my hands had remained intact. I had been spared by my personal relationship with baby Jesus. He was on my side, and we had an understanding. Yet seven more years at the school chipped away at this newfound relationship, and I came out of the nunnery an agnostic at best.

SEARCHING FOR A GOD OF MY OWN UNDERSTANDING

I left my hometown at the young age of seventeen and slowly found my way to the United States. My only possessions were a one-way ticket, a hundred-dollar bill, and a dream to get to San Francisco and wear some flowers in my hair. I arrived in California, the land of spiritual revolution, the Grateful Dead, Ram Das, and drugs. Looking to define myself I embraced several different spiritual disciplines but found that none really fit my personality. I was not likely to be a guru follower, I detested organized religion, and I did not like some of the strict hierarchies I found in several "enlightened" groups. If I wanted to get in touch with the original feelings I had felt that day as a five-year-old with baby Jesus, I had to build my own relationship with the Divine. All traditions pointed to the same methodology: prayer and meditation. I knew that prayers meant I would be asking God questions and that meditation meant I would be listening to the answers. Prayer and meditation, however, weren't enough. I had some scars to heal when it came to my relationship with the Divine, and I knew I needed to find a step-by-step guide to follow when life and all its challenges came screaming at me.

Years later, I joined a twelve-step program and started to find some answers. Through this program I learned that together with prayer and meditation, taking particular steps and using specific tools in a journey of self-discovery would allow me to stay on course in my life.[6] I was relieved that I was among people who would not impose their own idea of the Divine, and that I would be led to find my own definition and build my own relationship based on my commitment to honest living. Soon I realized that the purpose of prayer is not to ask my Higher Power to fix things for me, but rather to acknowledge and express my gratitude for all I have received. The purpose of meditation is to understand that Divine timing is different from my compulsive need to know and resolve things now. Finally, I realized that the keys to my serenity were patience and trusting that my Higher Power would take care of me.[7]

When I turned twenty-five and found myself pregnant with my first child, my journey of self-growth was fueled by a very specific goal: I was going to define my spiritual practice by first parenting myself and then parenting my unborn child. I resolved that my birthing experience had to be different from my mother's, different from what the American birthing industry was suggesting, different from all the negative images I was fed through the media, and different from the horror stories many women felt obligated to share with me once they saw my protruding belly. If I wanted to find what was right for me, I had to start at the beginning, my beginning.

MAKING PEACE WITH MY OWN BIRTH

I was born feet first, a breech baby. My mother trembled as she told me the story of my birth. With his naked hand, the doctor fished inside her womb to turn me around, performing a *version*[8] during my mother's late stage of labor. In agonizing pain, she kicked him in the face hard, hard enough to give him a black eye. Furious, the doctor left the delivery room, sought out my father, and asked him to decide which life he wanted to save. "Save my wife," my father responded, "we can always have another child."

As a consequence, my mother had gone through a great deal of pain and refused to see me for a couple of days, encouraged by a nurse who suggested she take the time to just rest and recuperate. She was reassured that her baby would be safely taken care of by the nurses in the nursery. What later came to light during a hypnosis session was that in the little plastic hospital crib in the cold and isolating nursery I had drawn a lifelong conclusion: "I don't deserve to be alive, my life is not important, my mom has abandoned me, I am unlovable."

That statement, that pact I made with myself at such an early age, deeply influenced the rest of my life. Recognizing it, voicing it, and allowing the feelings to surface during hypnosis as I carried my child in my womb, began a healing process that would allow me to live my pregnancy consciously and bring forth my baby at home and painlessly.

My hypnotherapist encouraged me to bring my adult-self with me into that nursery and parent my newborn-self, reassuring her that she not only had a right to be here in this world, for it was God's good pleasure to have her, but that she had the right to want and create the kind of birthing experience she truly deserved and desired. I did not know it at the time, but I had just declared the first of the Nine Basic Human Rights: the right to have and to be here.

MONTH

1

the right to be here and to have

I welcome the new life growing in my womb and affirm my right to have the birthing experience I desire and deserve. I declare the baby's right to be here on this planet and to have all that is necessary for its survival. I clearly set my intentions and prepare the fertile soil for the growth of a creative and confident human being. I let go of those people, places, and things that no longer serve me in my journey to find a new self, free from all the ties that bind me. I am grateful for all that is revealed. I let it go and so it is. Amen.

YOUR BABY NOW

The fertilized egg has made its seven-to-ten-day trip to the uterus, where it has implanted snugly into the endometrial surface. It is now called a blastocyst, and it has divided into two parts: one is forming the placenta, and the other will become the embryo. The two layers that make up the amniotic bag of waters are newly formed, and the very beginning of the connecting stalk that will become the umbilical cord has appeared. Until your placenta is fully functioning the yolk sac, now present, will feed your baby. The creative power has been unleashed and the life force has pure freedom of expression. The natural process of procreation is free from your logic, fear, and expectation. Your womb is gearing up. The energy required to provide for the new life is tremendous. Your biochemistry is changing rapidly. There is primordial joy: your womb has been called to do the job for which it was created.

You are no longer just a woman, you are becoming a mother. The transformation is subtle and irreversible. This new life form has not yet defined itself as an individual, and you are yet to fully conceive of yourself as a mother. Your partner, too, is going through a great transformation. No longer a "single" human being, he/she is becoming a parent. The miracle unfolds! It's time for welcomes. Come together with your loved one and read the following welcoming prayer to your baby as often as you can.

> *Welcome to the world, my love;*
> *we have been waiting for you.*
> *We are so happy you are here.*
> *You are the perfect expression of our love.*
> *We recognize your sacredness.*
> *We know you will teach us a great deal*

And we offer you all that we have,
All the love we can provide—unconditionally.
You will be free to be as special as you are meant to be.

THE FIRST CHAKRA

As I mentioned in the introduction, as we go through the nine months of gestation, we will focus on the corresponding energy centers, called *chakras* in the Eastern tradition.

The first chakra relates to our right to be here and to have what is necessary to survive and even thrive. In yoga, when we work on our first chakra—also referred to as the root chakra—we focus on our connection to the earth and our relationship with our culture and tribe's belief system, strengths, weaknesses, and fears. In its infancy, humankind was first and foremost focused on survival. We depended on the tribe for survival and sustenance. When we look upon the embryo in its first month of development, we see a beating heart that represents life struggling for its own survival, joined by a thin filament to a yolk sac that represents the fetus's sustenance. Dad's and Mom's chromosomes with all their data, including the data carried over from their own ancestry, have come together to form a unique expression of the Divine.

In the next eight weeks, all systems, organs, and tissues are put into place. If the embryo survives the next four to eight weeks, chances are the pregnancy will go all the way through to nine months.

How could anything so ephemeral as the mother's state of being have a lasting impact so very early, when there is just one or two or twelve cells?

The right to be here is the first basic human right. It is the root, or foundation, for all the work that lies ahead. Just as a plant grows tall and sturdy by having strong roots, we must nurture our relationship with Mother Earth and understand our ancestral and cultural roots. We must feel that we deserve to be in this world, that we are an inseparable part of it, yet that we can create our own life based on choices that are separate from our indoctrinations. In order to live a fulfilled life and bring forth a self-confident human being, we must declare our right to be here in this world and our right to have the birthing experience we choose.

IT IS YOUR CHOICE TO BE HERE

The notion of a life before conception can be found in many religious texts, spiritual teachings, and oral traditions. Documentation exists of children who have recalled another life altogether, one lived in another time and another place.

In their book *Cosmic Cradle: Souls Waiting in the Wings for Birth,*[9] Elizabeth Carman and her husband Neil Carman, Ph.D., compiled numerous accounts of individuals who, under hypnosis, recalled the realms where they existed before conception. Many of these people described choosing their parents and their life's purpose. Similarly, we find religious figures like Mother Teresa who declared, "I was born to serve God's poor," as if she believed her life's purpose had been decided even before she came into this world. Intuitive healer Carolyn Myss has written a book entitled *Sacred Contracts,*[10] in which she declares, "I believe that we each agree to the terms of our contract before entering the physical realm of this world."

Anthropologists tell us that some tribal traditions embrace the idea that the soul chooses its parent. Here is a wonderful story that describes how a tribe in Africa believes that it is the soul choosing the parent once the mother has opened herself to it. Jack Kornfield in Wayne Muller's *How, Then, Shall We Live?*[11] tells us this amazing story.

> . . . YOUR CHILDREN ARE NOT YOUR CHILDREN. THEY ARE THE SONS AND DAUGHTERS OF LIFE'S LONGING FOR ITSELF. THEY COME THROUGH YOU BUT NOT FROM YOU, AND THOUGH THEY ARE WITH YOU YET THEY BELONG NOT TO YOU.
>
> KAHLIL GIBRAN

There is a tribe in Africa where the birthdate of a child is counted not from when they've been born, nor from when they are conceived but from the day that the child was a thought in its mother's mind. And when a woman decides that she will have a child, she goes off and sits under a tree, by herself, and she listens until she can hear the song of the child that wants to come. And after she's heard the song of this child, she comes back to the man who will be the child's father, and teaches it to him. And then, when they make love to physically conceive the child, some of that time they sing the song of the child, as a way to invite it. And then, when the mother is pregnant, the mother teaches that child's song to the midwives and the old women of the village, so that when the child is born, the old women and the people around her sing the child's song to welcome it. And then, as the child grows up, the other villagers are taught the child's song. If the child falls, or hurts its knee, someone picks it up and sings its song to it. Or perhaps the child does something wonderful, or goes through the rites of puberty, then as a way of honoring this person, the people of the village sing his or her song. And it goes this way through their life. In marriage, the songs are sung, together. And finally, when this child is lying in bed, ready to die, all the villagers know his or her song, and they sing—for the last time—the song to that person.

Several Eastern and Western religious texts address the subject of life before conception, hinting at reincarnation. In the Koran, we find the following excerpts: "And you were dead, and He brought you back to life. And He shall cause you to die, and shall bring you back to life, and in the end shall gather you unto Himself" (2:28). The Bhagavad-Gita states, "Just as man discards worn out clothes, the soul discards worn out bodies and wears new ones" (2.22). Even Jesus refers to reincarnation in the following New Testament excerpt: "For all the prophets and the law have prophesied until John. And if you are willing to receive it, he is Elijah who was to come" (Matthew 11:13–14). And, "I say to you that Elijah has come already, and they did not know him. Then the disciples understood that he had spoken of John the Baptist" (Matthew 17:10–13). By identifying the Baptist as Elijah, who was dead at the time of John the Baptist, Jesus is talking about his spirit coming back as another. Buddha himself, who preferred not to discuss God or the soul, still preached that what he called the "ever-changing individual character" moves from birth to another birth, until all changing and becoming comes to an end.

Modern spiritual scholars have composed verses like this one by Sufi scholar Mansur al-Hallaj, attesting, "Like the herbage / I have sprung up many a time / On the banks of flowing rivers. For a hundred thousand years / I have lived and worked / In every sort of body."

So the sense that there is a life before life seems to be a recurring theme in humankind's belief system. When we realize this, we come to understand that the decision of our coming into this world was not merely based on our parents' intentional coming together or their accidental lovemaking, but a shared Divine choice we made with our parents. That choice was made either consciously or unconsciously, but nevertheless mutually.

If we agree with the possibility that our right to be in this world is based on our own choice and embrace this idea, we can make peace with the world around us and go on a journey to discover the purpose of this choice. What am I here for? What have I come to learn and/or teach?

As a young woman, I always felt the strong desire to be a mother. Since I can remember, I would fantasize about having a big family and caring for ten children. Yet, on the outside, my life as a performance artist traveling the world in a very bohemian fashion did not look like the right environment to bring a child into this world. Once I landed in the United States, I was overcome by a strong feeling that I had been here before, in another lifetime. I felt like I was home, and the desire inside my soul to be a mother increased exponentially. When I became pregnant with my first child, I decided to pierce the veil of illusion that time is divided into past, present, and future, and I went on a quest to answer the pressing questions of the reason for my existence and for my desire to become a mother.

CONCEPTION AND BIRTH OF MY SON

I was twenty-four years old, a performance artist, and married to a cartoon animator. After three years of marriage, I had decided to leave him because I wanted children and he didn't. I remember screaming at him and, in effect, to the universe: "I want a child, and if you don't want to be part of it, I am leaving this relationship!"

Six months after I separated from my husband, I found myself pregnant by a man I had just met. We had spent an amazing and loving weekend together and birth control could not prevent what fate had in store for me. After all, I had declared that I wanted a child and, as I have learned over and again, the universe's answer to such strong declarations is always "yes." The fact that I had wanted a child with my ex-husband and not with someone I had just met was the kind of detail the universe does not focus on. Once a desire is pronounced it seems the entire cosmos conspires to fulfill it.

My heart, body, and soul desperately wanted this child, but my practical and logical mind debated whether the circumstances were right for a baby. After the pregnancy test came back positive, confirming what my body had known all along, I gathered my courage and phoned the father, announcing: "We need to talk." He nervously replied, "Yes, I need to tell you something, too."

I later walked into his studio and blurted out my prepared speech. "Bruce," I said, "I'm pregnant. I understand if you don't want to have anything to do with this child. I think I want to have this baby, and you can participate in his life or not." Initially, he objected to having a baby this way, yet he also strongly rejected the idea that any child of his would live unaware of its own father. As I had anticipated, what he had planned to tell me was that we should break up. As he pleaded with me not to have the baby, to think about it a bit more, I ran out of the room, declaring histrionically, "You just don't get it, do you?"

Obviously, I wasn't getting it either. I had said that I wanted a child, but was I ready to be a single mother? Over the next few days, I found little refuge in my friends. Each girlfriend had a different opinion, and some only wanted to talk about what a great catch Bruce was. Asking my parents for counsel was out of the question. My Sicilian father's response would have been harsh, heaped with shame and disappointment. My mother would take this pregnancy as a personal affront: "Why are you doing this to me?"

The more I contemplated whether it was my right to have a child in these conditions, the more my resolve to have it dwindled. Meanwhile, the latest performance I was working on was centered on my mother's life during World War II and her involvement in the Italian partisan resistance. I created a collage of her stories and was writing a script in which I would play her. During rehearsals, playing my mother while being a mother sent me even further into confusion. I strongly believed, and still do, that there are no coincidences in one's life, but I needed someone to confirm all the signs that were hammering me over the head.

Living in California gave me the luxury to indulge in the most esoteric alternative sources of healing and self-discovery. I promptly made an appointment with a hypnotherapist and past-life reader. As soon as I arrived, her heart-warming smile put me at ease. She took me through a guided meditation. She said that I had all the answers within my soul; all I had to do was *remember*. As I entered a state of hypnosis, she reassured me that my questions would be answered by my guardian angels if I was willing to listen. I was skeptical—my cynical European heritage was still strongly embedded in me. Besides, I was not ready to hear what I had come to learn. Fear shut me down, and nothing seemed to come from our session. Disappointed, I decided to get a massage. I left the hypnotherapist's home and made an appointment with a masseuse. I thought, "Today I am not going to get any answers!" I was wrong.

I arrived for my massage, lay down on the table, closed my eyes, and finally relaxed. In a split second, I felt

I had been on the masseuse's table before, pampered by the same hands. Only I sensed it had been a long, long time ago. I tentatively opened my eyes to get my bearings and looked around. I recognized the room and heard her familiar voice. Yet something was very different.

I observed that the furniture was old and tattered. The massage table was now a rudimentary bed, and even the smells were different. I noticed the strong scent of her body, of musty wood, burning wax, and a faint smell of roses. Then, I saw a vase of pretty, pink roses on an antique chest, which had not been there when I first arrived.

My body, too, felt different, and as I looked down at my breasts, I blinked in disbelief. These were not my own, full, round breasts, but a smaller, perkier pair, and my skin had taken on a more sallow hue. I searched for the light source to see if a colored light bulb might have cast a yellow glow over the room. But I could not find a lamp or any electric lighting device. In fact, only candles illuminated the room.

I closed my eyes again, out of fear and in order to relax to her touch. I tried to calm myself down and understand where I was and *who* I was. A new vision came upon me, and this time I felt like a fly gazing into the room from a higher vantage point. I was both the person I was looking at and the observer.

I saw and felt myself in the body of a young woman who had been kidnapped and sold into prostitution during the California Gold Rush—a shy little Chinese girl, who had become pregnant on the job. I sensed her feelings of doom, fear, and longing. In this dimension, she and I were one. Her desperation was my own; neither she nor I knew what to do.

Her boss, the owner of her flesh, wouldn't allow her to keep the baby. She felt shame at what she had been forced to become. With no place to run and no family to turn to, she was utterly alone. Her friend was stroking her hair gently and lovingly, saying, "I will take care of you until the child is born. It happens all the time. The boss gets a lot of money for the babies born to his girls. You'll be all right!" To give her child, the only family she would know, to strangers who would probably use him as a laborer, was a cruel life sentence for the soul yet to be born. At that moment, I felt her overwhelming pain—she had no choice.

As happens in dreams, the next vision was a sort of fast montage of events. I saw her big belly, her carefree days in an isolated mountain cabin, other pregnant women's smiles, and I heard girlish laughter. In a tapestry of images and sensations, I witnessed the intensity of her labor and the love and compassion of the women around her. I felt her squatting, pushing, panting. Then I heard a final moan and a soft, gentle, baby cry.

A healthy, happy boy was there at her breast, feeding. She was not prepared for what blossomed inside her heart when the child was born. She never knew she was capable of such love. The love overwhelmed her, comforted her, and made her feel alive. I was one with this woman and felt all her emotions. Then, in a flash, back again in the witness role, I felt her anguish at the realization of what was to come. Her heart was invaded by a menacing cloud.

The midwife came to take her baby away. I took one last look into the baby boy's eyes and—I recognized him! I recognized the infant's expression, his deep-set eyes, and the echo of his adult features in his face. This baby resembled Bruce, the father of the child I was carrying in this life. I'd uncovered the unalterable connection between us, forged lifetimes ago.

When I finally woke up from the vision, I was sobbing and told the masseuse about the vision. She smiled. "It is not the first time that something like this has happened on my table. You have received the answer to your question," she said. The soul of the child I had given up in a past life had come back to fulfill our destiny together. Now all I had to do was follow my heart; all would be provided for. The answer appeared crystal clear: I could not give up the father of my child, or the child itself.

That night, I went to sleep and dreamed of a giant baby swimming in its large sack of amniotic fluids. As it lolled in the water and turned to face me, he—because it was a boy—opened his eyes and said, "My name is Azzurro, and you are going to have me."

The days that followed found me in a daze. Azzurro had no qualms about coming into the world. This celestial being growing inside of me had as much power as I did. When I told my son's father why I couldn't deny this child his place in the world, he surprised me by saying, "You are flipping crazy, but if you are going to have my baby, I come with the package!"

Since the amazing revelation on the masseuse's table, every moment, sign, and circumstance in my life has felt like a direct message from the Divine. I realized this pregnancy was a fantastic opportunity to come closer to my Creator, having now become a creator myself. Needing spiritual guidance, I sought readings that would help me shed light on my past, my belief system, and all that had been instilled into my psyche by my family, peers, and culture. I came to believe that bringing forth a child would give me a chance to birth a new, more conscious self. This was my life's lesson, this was my sacred contract. This child was not going to fix me; he was going to teach me how to fix myself. More precisely, this pregnancy would teach me how to enlist the Divine Mother to help me heal my past and re-tune my current behavior. Those sacred nine months offered a perfect opportunity to heal my soul.

Embracing and welcoming this new life, I began to consider how my experience of childbirth could be different from the one experienced by my mother. I went back to the hypnotherapist and relived my birthing experience. I made sure I healed the little girl inside and enlisted her help in creating the birthing experience she deserved, different from her own and instrumental for her healing.

Not knowing much about the how-tos of birthing, I went where most women go once they find out they are pregnant: the bookstore. The only book that spoke to me was Ina May Gaskin's *Spiritual Midwifery*.[12] Once I read it, I knew the book had been sent to me by the Mother herself. My son's birth was not going to be a medical event, but a sacred one. I took full charge of my pregnancy and the delivery of my child. I investigated alternative birthing methods, looked for a midwife willing to help me deliver at home, and read about natural childbirth from cultures around the world.

Through meditation, the power of creation that all women carry within had awakened in me. I modified an old Italian song into a welcoming message to my son. *"Azzurro il mio bambino è tutto Azzurro è bello per me . . ."* I sang Azzurro's song every day, as many times as I remembered. Azzurro's father created a little song of his own and began to sing it to my belly so our child would be familiar with his father's voice as well.

I continued my work as an artist, performing in galleries and theaters around the United States, using my art to delve deeply into my state and transforming my performances into a public birthing ritual. I worked and performed until the very last minute, wanting to learn as much as I could by staying conscious during my pregnancy and by sharing my feelings, emotions, and even my physical changes with an audience. I sought to share my happiness and the pride of my state. My pregnancy was an incredible emotional and transformational journey. Every day, I established a connection with the parts of my body that were changing and cradling my child. I also began exploring the places in my soul that needed healing, comforting, and spiritual growth.

On March 25, 1983, my water broke early in the afternoon as I was nesting. I called Bruce at work to let him know that this was going to be the day, but also that he had time to finish his work. I alerted the two girlfriends who had offered to be my doulas. I was excited and reveled in feelings of peace and self-confidence.

I began preparing the house. I checked all the home-birth supplies and changed my sheets. I ate small snacks throughout the evening and kept hydrated. I made my house into a sanctuary. I wanted to be alone at first, to commune with God and Azzurro and visualize the approaching birthing experience.

As I listened to soothing music, I went inside my body and communicated with all the parts that were going to partake in this ritual. I talked to my cervix and connected her to mental images of a blossoming flower gently opening at the coming of dawn. I massaged my perineum and told it to be prepared to stretch and allow my son's head to pass through. I caressed my inner thighs and told them I needed their support in my squatting. I asked the Divine Mother to come into my humble abode and hold my hand and show me how to fulfill my vocation as a woman.

By seven o'clock, Bruce had come home. He took command of the ship: I was to concentrate on the waves of labor. Bruce helped relieve the pressure on my lower back by constantly massaging it. Azzurro was in a posterior presentation, pushing on my back all through the labor. We kept silent most of the time. By ten that evening, my girlfriends arrived to help. By midnight, my contractions were regular at five minutes apart, and Nina, our midwife, came over. When she checked me, I was eight centimeters dilated and 100 percent effaced. She suggested a warm relaxing bath.

The bath was glorious; I was able to envision myself as a giant whale riding the waves of contractions. When it was time to push (and here I began calling this phase hugging the baby out), Nina suggested I clench the handle of the bedroom door, squatting with my legs on each side, using gravity to help the baby down the birth canal. After pushing this way for about an hour, I lay on my bed and my girlfriends sat on either side of me. Placing one foot on the shoulder of each of them while holding onto their arms, I pushed for another forty minutes. My dear son's head emerged. Bruce and Nina readied to catch the baby. As he was born, Azzurro looked directly into his father's eyes. Bruce caught him and gently placed this magical bundle onto my chest.

At that point, my renewed soul collided and merged with Azzurro's. Motherhood arrived in search of me. I don't know exactly where it came from. Was it my heart or my womb? There were no voices, no words, nor silence, but as Pablo Neruda says, "from paradise I was summoned." The deepest love sprouted inside me directly from the branches of the tree of life. Following the potent waves of the creative ocean, I returned victorious, holding the fruit of my loins.

My mouth had no way with words. My eyes were blinded by Azzurro's beauty, and something awakened in my soul. I began rambling, uttering the first faint sounds—without substance, pure nonsense, pure love. Then I heard the sound of heaven: my son's first breath, his cry, his declaration of existence on this earth. So I sang his song to him. Drunk from the experience, I felt myself part of the universe; "I wheeled with the stars, soared with the wind."

I cannot tell you I didn't feel the pressure of birth. I cannot tell you I was cosmically anesthetized, but what I can tell you is that my concentration and communion with the Divine Mother was such that I felt as if I was in another dimension. Azzurro's birth was very intense as he was in a posterior presentation. It took months of introspection and realization to come to the conclusion that indeed I could not call what I felt painful.

Our lovely son was born at home on Saturday, March 26, 1983, at 1:39 a.m., weighing eight pounds. I took a shower while the bed was cleaned and prepared for the night. Bruce, Azzurro, and I slept peacefully, cuddling in our bed.

I breastfed Azzurro for one year. Every time he cried, I picked him up and sang his song. As if by magic, he would immediately quiet down and revel in my familiar voice. To this day, Azzurro, my daughter Natascia, and I continue to share a special bond and, at times, as we cuddle I still sing them their special songs.

THE RIGHT TO HAVE THE BIRTHING EXPERIENCE YOU DESIRE

What I have learned is that before we can communicate with our child and welcome him into this world, we need to welcome ourselves and visit our child-self in our mother's womb. The first step is to revisit your own birthing experience. Ask your mother to tell you what she went through, how she felt. If your mother is no longer alive, you might want to go to a hypnotherapist and have a few sessions until you remember your own entrance into this world. You can also go into a meditative state on your own and bring yourself back to the beginning of your life, but it is not advisable to do this work alone. At least share your experience with a trusted friend. If there is healing to be done, bring your adult-self with you on this journey of rebirthing. As you go back into the memory, use your adult-self to heal any wounds that might still be festering deep inside your unconsciousness. It is never too late to give yourself the welcome you deserve and to affirm your fundamental right to have the birthing experience you desire.

Sara's Story

Sarah's first child had been posterior and she had experienced excruciating back labor pain and had opted for an epidural. She came to me late in her second pregnancy, seeking some hypnotherapy sessions to help her approach this birthing experience differently. We decided that for our first session we would revisit her own birthing experience.

Under a deep state of hypnosis, she recalled that her mother did not know the sex of her child prior to the birth. Her mother's drug-free labor had been long and painful, for Sarah herself had been in the posterior position. Once her mother had been told she had given birth to a baby girl, she exclaimed "Oh no, a girl! How unlucky my little one; you too will have to experience this horrible pain in childbirth!" Newly born and desperately needing her mother's love, attention, and reassurance, Sarah immediately made an unconscious pact with herself: she would do just as her mother had told her. Her only desire was to please her mom and in that attempt as a little girl she had resolved that if she was going to have the same painful birthing experience her mother had, she would gain her respect.

Once Sarah came out of the hypnotic state, she realized she had been totally unaware of this pact. Within seconds of having been born, Sarah's primal right to be here had become subconsciously attached to her duty to have the same birthing experience as her mother had. We worked together a few more times before her second child's birth. Each time, she discovered how that original pact had been the root of other feelings of unworthiness, feelings which had sprung from her desperate need for her mother's approval. In reviewing some of her past, Sarah realized that growing up, no matter how hard she had tried, she just couldn't please her mother. This need to be recognized and loved by her mom had taken over during her last pregnancy and birth, and she had fulfilled her promise to have a painful posterior delivery. Would this new, deep knowledge be sufficient for Sarah to break her own pact now and have a different birthing experience?

As we continued working together, we saw that despite the realization of what her pact had been, adult Sarah was still very attached to pleasing her mother. She often complained that her mother preferred her sister-in-law and was not willing to give time to Sarah. Even though she was beginning to be aware of her patterns, she was still focusing on comparing her mother's love and dedication to her brother and his wife. Our meetings were often dedicated to discussing her feelings of anger over something her mother did that felt unjust to her.

When her labor began, all her good, rational intentions disappeared and, despite her resolve to labor at home, Sarah called her mother to care for her first-born daughter and rushed to the hospital. Adult Sarah abdicated, and her child-self took over the difficult job of wrangling the waves of contractions. Once I joined her, she did not want to be touched by anyone, she did not want to be talked to, and when I attempted hypnosis, she screamed, "That's not working for me! I don't want to hear it!" I had no way of reaching her; she had built a wall around herself so that even with her best intentions, all that she had planned before the birth went out the window as the child-self took over and made all the decisions.

Even though her second baby was not posterior, her body remembered and focused on the back pain, and that memory sent her mind into an unreachable, unconscious place. As soon as she got an epidural, Sarah was finally relaxed and able to come back to her adult-self. Her labor progressed quickly, and within two hours she successfully hugged her baby out. Her confidence and well-being came back as soon as her baby girl was placed on her bosom.

When I went to visit her at home later on, we discussed the birth. She told me she did not know exactly what had happened, but remembered her mother telling her, "It will be OK to get an epidural if you really need one." Once again, her mother's permission had talked to her child-self, and she did what she had been given permission to do.

In reviewing the birth, Sarah could say with confidence that she was proud of the outcome of this birth, in spite of the epidural. This birth had been different from her first one. This time, she had stepped into consciousness once it was time to welcome her baby into the world (which she had not done with her first child), and had been able to witness her process, even though she had not been able to stop her child-self from taking over. She needed to heal her programming and became willing to do it. Upon my departure, she said, "Baby number three will be different."

In order to have a different birthing experience from the one our mother had, or thinks we should have, we need to become conscious of our programming so that we may make changes that will be in unison with our deepest desires.

THE RIGHT TO HAVE: PROGRAMMING

Change comes with learning, but the most constructive transformation comes with unlearning. It's important to realize that our old ways of thinking are a big part of our future success. What stories have you heard? What beliefs have been instilled in you in the arena of birthing, motherhood, and pain management? In short, what is the birthing blueprint of your unconscious mind?

Your birthing blueprint consists of your thoughts, feelings, and actions in relation to labor and delivery. We have all been conditioned by our families, cultures, religious leaders, the medical industry, and the media. There are three primary ways of conditioning: oral programming, imitation, and experiential.

Oral Programming

What you've heard and have been told while growing up can color your experiences of today. A baby's survival depends on his family. All he learns comes from the village he inhabits. As the old African adage says, "It takes a village to raise a child."

In order to stand by your right to have your wishes come true, you must first shed the skin you've inherited from your family of origin, environment, culture, religion, and tradition. All the hand-me-downs you have been wearing represent the rules you have learned: what is right and what is wrong; what is accepted and what is not; what is the norm and what is your truth. If you are not in charge of your own thoughts, your decisions, and your opinions, someone else is. That's when you abdicate all resolution to your care provider, instead of participating in the decision-making. In doing so, you choose what is the norm: what others tell you and what is deemed best by someone else.

Imitation

What you have seen and learned to imitate will be your current default behavior. Have you noticed how at times you are thinking your mom's thoughts, or you have taken over your dad's opinion and even mannerisms? Our default behaviors come from imitation. Default behaviors are behaviors that come up when you are in a crisis. Thus, when you are in the midst of a fight, you may imitate exactly what your mother or father would do or say. Imitation becomes particularly noticeable in parenting patterns. When a child misbehaves and the parent is at the end of her rope, she often repeats the same actions and delivers the same punishment her mother did. In a crisis, our most primitive brain, the one responsible for our survival mechanisms, gets activated and our behaviors become automatic. In this way, especially if the experience is new, we react the only way we know how to—namely, in the manner we have seen others react. This is one of the reasons parents who were abused as children sometimes abuse their own children. These people live an unconscious life and don't heal the past. If we want to stand on our own, we need to look into our indoctrination that comes from imitation, and we need to learn new behaviors and new solutions to the crises that arise.

EXPERIENCE

In modern society, we are no longer surrounded by a large extended family as we were hundreds of years ago when we lived in villages. As a result, we are likely to have witnessed birth only through the media. On TV, we commonly hear that birth is a long and painful event, that the hospital is the sane place to have our child, and that the use of drugs to numb labor is truly the modern way to manage birth. Movies have shown us images of laboring women screaming in agony and insulting their husbands as they demand pain medication. The images of birth are routinely of a masked doctor who delivers the baby and shows him to the mother for a moment before he hands him off to a nurse. The baby gets cleaned, checked, poked, weighed, measured, and finally wrapped in several blankets and a hat before being returned to his mother in the best case scenario, or simply shown to her before getting whisked away to the nursery where more tests are done. The baby is often abandoned, allowed to scream ("it's good for his lungs," affirms the nurse at the nursery), pacified with a plastic sucker, and even fed artificial baby food through a bottle, for the mother needs to rest. Though these scenes might make us angry or even laugh, the power of the big screen and the vividness of these images make us believe that this is the norm and that this is what will happen to us.

What you have been told by your family, your friends, and your society might not reflect what you want for yourself and your child, but you need to inform yourself of the alternatives that are available and then let go of your old ways, old ideas, and old programming.

If you want to stand for your right to have a painless and natural childbirth, you must alter your programming. You cannot change other people's opinion, you cannot modify what happened in the past, and you cannot alter what the media shows, but you can take certain steps to divert your life course.

The first element of all transformation is awareness. Begin by writing down your birth-related programming, modeling, and the specific incidents you have witnessed in your family history. Become conscious and watch yourself. Observe your thoughts, your beliefs, your fears, your habits, your actions, and your inactions. Put yourself under a microscope.

Linda's Story

My mother had three Cesarean sections, my sister had two. I had a suspicion that none of these was medically necessary, and so I wanted very badly to have a vaginal delivery. So much so that I opted not to alert my doctor or my birth coach and best friend when I went into labor. I was waiting to progress on to the real moments of labor before showing up at the hospital.

A few hours later, after my water had broken, still waiting for *real* labor to prompt me, I checked in with my coach. She convinced me to see my doctor, who wanted to start an immediate C-section. I refused, and the doctor angrily sent me away. Later that day, my coach and I went to the emergency room, where I ended up having my baby vaginally. My best friend was right there with me through thick and thin, along with a wonderful resident who had every reason to think I was a nutcase, as I arrived unannounced at the ER.

I still feel lucky that my assumption that I'd be able to have a vaginal delivery worked out. I am grateful for the blessings of all the people who lined up to support me and my baby in the ER and afterward.

Instinctively, women know what kind of birth they want, yet at times they fight with themselves and others over their right to have the kind of birthing experience they prefer. Despite their initial impulse, they may even begin to question their own decisions. This lack of trust in our instincts often comes from a sense of not belonging. Maybe we were told we were a mistake our parents made, or maybe dad wanted a boy and not a girl. In the case of Linda, she was told by her doctor she was destined to follow her family's Cesarean history. She had to fight hard and go against other people's judgments to obtain the kind of birth she knew she could have. After you have taken the first steps to become aware of your indoctrination and you come to a place where you own your right to be here in this world, you can turn your attention to your right to have the birthing experience you deserve and desire. To have something new, you must let go of the old.

CHANGE

As a river flows, it is always renewing itself. It is ever-changing, cradling new life in its clear and fresh waters. A flowing river is a source of considerable energy, responsible for transforming its own shape and form. Be that river and purify yourself from all debris that has accumulated in your past. Cleanse yourself of any person, place, or pact that does not contribute to your new state of serenity and replenishment. Instead of viewing the past like a stagnant pond, realize that the water keeps moving, forever changing. Although we may not be able to erase what has happened, we have the power to transform the way we experience it. We may need to make room for the new by letting go of the old. Sometimes we need to say goodbye and release our old ways, old friends, old habits, old life, old beliefs, and old thoughts. It is not easy, but it is necessary.

Immerse yourself in a warm tub, close your eyes, and feel the ever-changing water surround you. As the ever-flowing water of the river clears the debris and purifies itself, prepare yourself for the ritual of letting go of all that no longer serves you. Imagine long, silver strands that connect you to those people, places, and things that are no longer acceptable in your life. Ask your Higher Power to give you shears of light, and with loving thoughts begin to sever all ties that bind you. As you do this, send forgiveness, love, and good wishes, and let go peacefully.

You are protecting yourself and your child; you are making room. You might need to do this paring more than once before you feel you have truly let go. Don't fear. It is OK. Cutting ties with those who encumber you doesn't mean you will never see these people again or never talk to them again. With this spiritual pruning, you begin to learn to release the negative hold they have on you. You are making room for your baby, clearing away knots that shadow your life. Trust in your Higher Power, which does not close a door unless another is ready to be opened. As you come out of the clear water restored and renewed, it time to connect to Mother Earth.

CONNECTING WITH MOTHER EARTH: AN EXERCISE

If you are familiar with yoga, you are familiar with the child's pose. Begin on your knees, sit on bent legs, and let your body fall forward, forehead on the floor, while your arms are stretched alongside you. Close your eyes and imagine you are a seed, deeply embedded into the earth. Take a deep breath in and allow yourself to visualize what it would be like to sprout tiny roots into the soil and slowly emerge into the beautiful plant you are meant to become. Get into the feeling of being a seed growing toward its future.

Cherish every moment of being a seed, and make sure that each element of your sprouting body supports the rest of the growth. Don't be impatient and raise your head above the ground too fast, knowing that your stem is too long for the weight of the first two leaves, or that a brisk wind would crush your small body. Allow yourself to grow slowly, just as nature designed. What kind of plant are you? Are you a tree, or a vegetable that brings joy to someone's lips? Are you a fragrant flower that will inspire a smile? Ground yourself in your soil and take in its nourishments.

Immerse yourself once a day for the next seven days into

this feeling of being a child seed. Each day will bring you new insight and bring you closer to the seed that is sprouting inside your womb. This exercise can help you commune with your embryo in its early stage, and you may have an understanding of what your embryo is going through.

IF YOU WANT SOMETHING, YOU MUST FIRST BELIEVE YOU CAN HAVE IT

Can you imagine a little chick inside its egg complaining about its surroundings, wishing for a larger egg with more yolk, more albumen, more space? Its desire is limited by its narrow imagination. The chick is afraid to break through the only possession or home it thinks it has, unaware that once it smashes through the thin shell of its perceived boundaries, an entire world appears. In the realm of nature, this sounds like a ridiculous scenario.

However, some people are like that imaginary chick, living as if they are surrounded by a tight shell. All they dare want is what they believe is reasonably obtainable: a normal life, a healthy baby, a reasonable income, and a roof over their head. These people often feel stuck in life, but they do not dare want more. They may complain a lot, but they often say, "I am reasonable. Not everyone can be rich and happy and have all they want. As long as I am healthy and safe, I don't really need that much. If everyone else is having an epidural, why should I be any different?"

Observe how in nature there are no doubts. The chick breaks through the egg; the baby comes out of the womb, curious and filled with an instinctual desire to daydream, explore, and expand. Children are born with tremendous imaginations. Yet as they grow, social, cultural, and familial notions are imposed, and their circle of availability is defined. Here are the stories they are sometimes told:

If your parents are dirt poor, you might as well not dream big, for you are probably going to end up like them. If you're a minority and come from the ghetto, you'll probably live a poor life. If you are white and lead a privileged life, you cannot be a hip-hop star. If you are short, you cannot play basketball. If you have a learning disability, you'll never amount to anything. If you are going to have a baby, you'll experience unmanageable pain and should go to the hospital and get some drugs to numb it.

By the time a child is an adult, she is surrounded by an invisible sphere that limits her achievable goals. Her circle of availability is made up of all the things she perceives as reachable; a glass of water is within reach, but a painless childbirth is unobtainable.

One way to expand your circle of availability is to realize that all you desire already exists. Kids from the hood have grown up to become business tycoons, there are white hip-hop stars and successful basketball players short in stature but grand in performance. Most important, however, is that studies have shown that forty thousand women each year in the United States alone experience a painless childbirth. As long as one person can break through her imposed circle of availability, we can all do it. Here's an exercise that can help you do just that.

EXERCISE

Get a large board and make a collage of mementos that remind you of all your achievements. Call it the Achievement Board. Take photos of trophies you've won in sports competitions, use business cards from jobs you've had and are proud of, copies of grants you have received, images of the car you finally purchased. Add photos of your wedding, of your first born, or of the dream vacation you had. Use anything, big or small, that will remind you of your dreams that have come true. Next, take several 4 x 6 cards and write on each card something you want to accomplish. Don't forget to include "a painless childbirth." Place these cards on your desk or your nightstand next to the Achievement Board. Start each day by looking at what you have achieved. Get into the feeling of each accomplishment and the sense of satisfaction it brought you. When you are brimming with excitement from what you have already accomplished, look at one of the cards that represent your future goals and transfer those feelings onto that new goal. Now close your eyes and act as if you have already accomplished this goal. Stay in this state for as long as you can. The more you believe that you have accomplished and obtained your heart's desires, the more you will be sure to make it happen. This is what people call the Law of Attraction.

THE LAW OF ATTRACTION

You attract into your life what you think about, whether wanted or unwanted. The Law is neutral, and it always says yes. Thus, if you say you don't want to be sick, it brings sick to you. The law only works in the positive. It does not distinguish from want or don't want, it focuses on the object of your desire. Thus, if you don't want to be sick, you must focus on how healthy you are or want to be. All forms of matter and energy are attracted to that which is of a like vibration. You are a living magnet. Energy attracts like energy. So if you worry about not being able to take the pressure of the contractions, you won't be able to do exactly that. You are attracting the energy of fear and fueling it. If you act in confidence, you'll simply get more confidence. Everything draws to itself that which is like itself. If you state from the very beginning that you will have a painless child-birth and you say it until your entire being believes it, you will attract it.

THE RIGHT TO HAVE A PAINLESS CHILDBIRTH

Many of my clients state that they have experienced a natural and painless childbirth. When I say painless, please understand, I don't mean you will not feel anything. What you will feel is a lot of pressure; you will feel the might of creation come through you. Pain, however, is associated with something gone wrong. Childbirth is a lot of hard work, and the sensations that accompany it are very strong, but there is nothing wrong with labor.

Labor is what happens when a baby comes into this world. Remember, unless complications occur, you are not a patient; you are a healthy, birthing mother using the hospital facility to bring your child into this world. Labor comes one minute at a time, and if you focus on managing that one minute, you will be able to conquer it.

Stay open to all possibilities. You can have a painless childbirth even if for some reason you need an emergency Cesarean delivery. We are blessed with modern technology, great medicine, and amazing doctors who are standing by ready to help us in the moment of need. We embrace all births and we take charge of our own as we stay open to whatever happens. By choosing a supportive team and a supportive hospital, you can rest assured that nothing will be done without your informed consent, or without due cause. Painlessness is a state of well-being that embraces body, mind, and spirit. It is your right to have a painless childbirth, especially if you think you deserve one.

DESERVING GREATNESS

At times, we fear success more than we fear failure. After all, most of us are familiar with failure. It is not that unnatural to endure failure or to foresee it. But what of success? Do we know it as well? Do we even deserve it? Are we worthy of it? Do we have a right to have it?

As the seed is genetically coded to become a splendid flower, and the embryo is coded to become a precious baby, you are spiritually coded to be a superb expression of the Mother God. The magnificence that you are is the gift you have come to give the world. You deserve to be great. Your greatness does not belong to you alone. Your greatness is here to serve others. The closer you get to God, the closer you get to your natural talent to help and protect others. You are one with the Divine Mother; you are the celestial receptacle for God's miracle—to unfold, expand, and become a perfect symbol of Mother's love for us all.

Humbly accept your greatness, and humbly rejoice in the glory of life. Each and every action in your life is your ministry. Motherhood is your ministry. Being a business-woman, a pilot, an engineer, or an artist is your ministry. Being a wife is your ministry, being a friend is your ministry, being a daughter and a sister is your ministry. Share the glory, share your gifts, and share the love.

If you embrace the silence and allow your own true nature, your God nature, to come through, you will slowly feel the power and knowledge of the Mother shine through you. You will stand with your own thoughts, ideas, and intention for this pregnancy and the birth of the baby. You will be able to help the embryo feel at this very early stage your own clarity about your life's purpose. You have come here to share a gift only you can give; to be someone only you can be; to add something very special to this world. Maybe your life's purpose is as simple as having a relationship with your child in the years to come. Maybe you were built for greatness and are destined to change our world as we know it. Whatever the reason for your being and for your baby's being, show him your natural right to have and to be here.

Shed all that you have absorbed through the collective consciousness, its strength, its fears, its beliefs, and its response pattern. Birth a new self, a child of wonder rediscovering each and every moment as your first. Today, taste an orange, see the ocean, smell the rain as it falls to the ground, as if you were doing it for the very first time.

When the old is shed, feel the present moment. Know that whatever comes forth, it can be handled, for you have all the knowledge of the Divine universe within you. All you need to do is allow it to act through you.

A Closing Prayer

Welcome to the world, sweet baby. You are a magnificent expression of the Divine. We recognize you and we thank God for you. We will teach you love and trust by showing you how we love and trust each other. We will be open and honest with you. We hear you, we see you, and we love you immensely. We give you permission to be different from us, to be like us, to be all that we are, more or less than we are, and we encourage you to explore your own unique path and forms of expression. We have full confidence in you; we know you can do anything you really want to do. If you fall down, ask for our help, and we will support you while you learn the tools and skills of self-support. You are a magnificent and beautiful creature, and we are honored and ready to be your parents. While you are establishing your own boundaries, we will set limits for you, we will enforce those limits, and at times, because we love you, we will say no. In addition to, and sometimes in spite of your actions and behavior, we will love you for who you are. The warmth of your spirit that shines in your eyes glows in your smile that radiates from your heart. Listen to your own inner voice, for it is God's voice that resides in your own innermost spirit. In you, dear child, lies the power of peace and joy for the entire universe.

MONTH

2

the right to feel and the right to want

I declare my right to feel and to express my feelings as I learn to be compassionate with myself and others. I unleash my dreams, releasing the limitations of my own thoughts and my own perceptions. I embrace this child growing inside my womb, respect where she comes from, and where she is destined to go. I accept the teachings she brings to me and feel the sacredness of our connection. I declare my right to want the birthing experience I deserve, and as I do so, I give life to a person in harmony with the world. I am grateful and filled with joy for what I feel and want, and I simply let it be. And so I am, and so it is. Amen

YOUR BABY NOW

Proportionally speaking, your baby's head is quite big, due to the rapid growth of the brain. The upper limbs resemble paddles. The heart begins to separate into four chambers, and blood is circulating throughout the body. The intestines are forming within the umbilical cord, and they will later migrate back into the abdominal cavity. In the next few days, foot plates, with the beginnings of toe rays, will appear. The external ears are now present. Your baby is now about the size of a cherry. The cells that become either testes or ovaries arrive, but there is no obvious sign of gender yet. Muscle contractions are beginning, but these early movements are not yet perceptible to you. In this stage, the child is beginning to define its limits and boundaries, growing limbs and fingers to touch and feel the world outside itself.

YOUR BODY: MORNING SICKNESS AND TIREDNESS

This morning, you just don't feel right. In fact, you feel awful, uncomfortable in your skin, tired, and even a bit depressed. Congratulations! You are pregnant and your body is working harder in these first months to build the baby's internal organs. So here are a few suggestions for the nausea blues:

- Keep crackers at the side of your bed.
- Don't wake up and get going. Rather, first open your eyes, munch on a cracker, and go through your daily gratitude list.
- Don't drink with your meals, as this sometimes increases nausea, but drink plenty between meals.
- Sip tea or carbonated waters (no sodas), and try fresh lemonade.
- Stay away from excessive motion or loud noises.

- Play some quiet classical music when you wake up. Tension is directly connected to your stomach. Even a wrist-band for sea-sickness can really help!
- Ginger can do wonders. You can get it as candy, ginger pills, or ginger tea with lots of honey and a little lemon.

When at work, try to get in a few power naps or intentional breaks. Close your eyes and take one deep breath. As you exhale, let go of the last conversation you had and the thought of what you need to do next. Simply concentrate your attention on your breath. With each inhale visualize a comforting glow surrounding your budding baby, and with each exhale all the tension and all the worries melt away. All you need is a series of two to three breaks in your day and you will feel rested and much stronger.

If you don't have minutes, then take seconds; just call it the ten-second power nap. Quantity is a human experience; quality is Divine. As long as you can completely free yourself from the past and the future and truly be in the moment, a break of any duration can be beneficial.

THE SECOND CHAKRA

The second chakra relates to our right to feel. It is also called the partnership chakra. It sits under our belly button and the physical organs that surround this area. Thus, the uterus that holds our baby is ruled by this chakra. At a spiritual and healing level, it represents our relationships with other people. Sometimes this is exhibited by the need we have to control people, places, and things in order to feel safe. As the embryo extends its arms and fingers to touch the other, we are asked to look deeply into our feelings and find out where they come from. Rudolf Steiner, in the early 1900s, taught that, "During pregnancy, the mother's joy and pleasure are the forces that provide her baby with perfect organs."[13] As we become conscious of their origins, we can zero in on the true nature of our desires and formulate what we want. The lesson to learn relates to acknowledging, honoring, and respecting the other while we respect, honor, and acknowledge ourselves.

THE RIGHT TO FEEL

All our actions are born from feelings. Whether the feelings come from our conscious or subconscious mind, they lead us to take action. When we feel unsafe, we choose actions that are protective, limited, cautious, and non-expansive. When we feel confident, we stretch ourselves to reach goals that others might think are impossible. In order to become conscious of our feelings to manage our reactions, we need to discover where they come from.

For many years, medical scientists defined a baby as physical matter, especially brain matter, that had no ability to register or process memory, learning, trauma, emotion, or any truly human experiences until months after birth. In 1980, a study on prenatal stimulation was conducted in Caracas, Venezuela, under the direction of psychologist Beatriz Manrique.[14] The results stirred interest in the psychology community. Six hundred families, divided into experimental and control groups, were involved in a project that tested the babies for six years following their prenatal program. These studies proved what few believed prior to 1980: (1) that babies in the womb are alert, aware, and attentive to activities involving voice, touch, and music; (2) that babies benefit from these activities by forming stronger relationships with their parents and their parents with them, making for better attachments and better birthing experiences; and (3) that these babies tend to show precocious development of speech, fine and gross motor performance, better emotional self-regulation, and better cognitive processing.[15]

If babies are aware and alert while in the womb, then our emotions can create an environment that can be perceived as either pleasant and supportive of learning or unpleasant, suppressant, and geared to protect the status quo. Once aware of their influences on the unborn babies, many of my clients are in fear of any strong negative emotion. They feel the pressure to be happy and serene and become almost paralyzed by it, afraid of doing something wrong and often angry at those who take their apparent serenity away. It's better to realize that we are here to teach our children how we deal with whatever comes up in life, not to shield them completely. As a mother, it is your responsibility to teach your child how to resolve situations, not evade them.

FEELINGS INVENTORY

People facing the same situation can have diametrically different emotions. There are two basic feelings—good and bad—and two ways to confront and assimilate what happens in our lives. When a conflict arises and we feel bad, we can either learn from it, bettering ourselves and our lives, or we can consider it a challenge and perpetuate the conflict by reacting to protect ourselves and by attempting to preserve what we believe to be right. In so doing, we forfeit the chance to grow and learn.

As a parent, your responsibility is to teach your child by example. Therefore, you have to learn how to express and share your feelings so that you may teach your baby to do the same safely.

Dina's Story

Dina came to see me because she could not stop raging at her mother every time they discussed her desire to have a homebirth. Angry, upset, and depressed, Dina would isolate herself, which made things much worse. While she felt confident that her decision was a good one, she knew her reactions to any criticism were exaggerated. She kept telling me, "I hate it when people tell me I'm wrong. It feels like a kettle inside my stomach is about to burst!"

I suggested that she close her eyes and recall the emotions she felt whenever her mother recommended anything about her pregnancy. Once deeply settled into those feelings, I guided her through the following Feelings Inventory Exercise.

1. *When was the very first time you felt this feeling? Go back as far as you can remember, and describe in detail what happened and how old you were.*

Dina recalled that she had had a learning disability as a child. One of her earliest memories, before anyone realized she was dyslexic, was of her fifth grade teacher telling her that she did not work hard enough. She was labeled as lazy and sent home with a note to this effect. Her mom punished Dina for being a lazy girl who would not amount to anything unless she worked harder.

2. *How did you feel as a result of what happened?*

She responded that her world had fallen apart. She felt alone and unlovable. She worked hard to show everyone that she was not lazy, yet no matter how hard she tried, she just couldn't excel. It took years for her parents to realize that she had a learning disability and, by that time, Dina had resolved not to trust anyone.

3. *What did you come to believe about yourself as a result of this event and these feelings?*

Dina felt her mother did not love her, since she would not believe her. The grownups were all telling her she was lazy, but knowing she wasn't, Dina concluded that she must be stupid or slow. It was surprising to the adult woman now in my office to uncover that she had such low self-esteem. She truly thought she had a higher opinion of herself. When I asked Dina the question above, she revealed that she'd come to believe, "I am stupid, slow. I am unworthy and unlovable."

When we go into labor, the unconscious mind takes over and we often revert to feelings and behaviors that come from our child-self. This has been depicted in several movies in the form of a perfectly sweet woman who, in labor, turns into a raging monster as she insults her husband and appears unmanageable. While this depiction of women is only intended to make you laugh, there is an important message we can extract from these scenes. If we don't heal the unconscious mind, it might show up and rule the outcome of our birthing experience.

4. *Now, look at the present. How do those old beliefs color your life today?*

Dina began to see how even today, she is overly cautious about everything and everyone. She was known to rant and rave at work if asked to clarify the smallest matter, or whenever anyone dared to hint that she might be wrong about anything. She chose to be a saleswoman because she simply could not work in an office. Her boss only retained her despite her temper because she made good money for the company. Dina had married late, as it was very difficult for her to trust any man that came into her life and to trust that her marriage would last.

5. *Finally, consider this: How would a loving person truly describe you? How would your Higher Power want to hear you portray yourself?*

When it came to answering this question, tears began streaming down Dina's cheeks. She realized that while she had been hard on others, she had been especially hard on herself. The person she trusted least was herself. Feeling constantly attacked and needing always to protect herself, she restored to isolating. This exercise had shed some light into her darkness. I suggested she come up with an affirmation to recite every morning and night, and especially every time she felt that "kettle" inside her gut about to burst.

Dina's affirmation was, "I am lovable and intelligent. I am a good and capable mother. I am safe. I trust in my innate ability to know what is right for me and my child."

When we met the following week, things had gotten a bit better. Dina told me that she now felt she knew why she was getting so mad, and that often she'd just close her eyes and repeat the affirmation to cool down. She had also had a long and heartfelt conversation with her mother about what had happened and why she was still reacting this way. Dina laughed because during the conversation with her mom, she had to repeat the affirmation to herself at least ten times. She had been able to go through an entire exchange with her mom without having a big fight. The healing had begun.

HOW YOU FEEL ABOUT ME IS NONE OF MY BUSINESS

We often enter into conflict to protect ourselves. Most people's feelings are aligned with their need to be right and to be understood. We feel bad about criticisms only when we believe them to be true. If someone called you an eggplant, you would laugh it off or call them insane. But if they said you were fat or stupid or unlovable, that may strike a deep chord. If deep inside you agree with the criticism, you'll become defensive and angry and lash out at the person who has offered it. Thus, we do not react solely to the words, but also to an old core belief about ourselves that the words evoke. If you agree with the critical assessment, it will hurt you; if you don't, you will be able to dismiss it and even look at the person that has expressed it with compassion. Lashing out and insulting someone is a defense mechanism. When you hear a particular criticism that resonates, deal with the pain by considering it a signal to humbly look within and see what truth may lie there. You might not agree with what you're hearing, but attend to the message rather than focusing on the messenger. If the universe is repeatedly sending the same theme through different people, pay attention. Stay open and learn from each situation. The ultimate act of love and courage is self-examination. To engage in conflict with others requires far less strength of character.

FEELINGS SHARED

One common way we protect ourselves and others is by minimizing or hiding what we really feel. Some of us have been taught that our feelings are wrong and have been told: "Stop crying. There is nothing to cry about! Stop that silly laugh! Wipe that grin off your face right now, young lady! I don't appreciate that tone of voice, it is just not ladylike!"

Another defensive strategy is just the opposite: maximizing. People who employ this tactic let everyone know how they feel with unbridled self-expression. They yell, rant, or simply pout to show how indignant and angry they are. These people are no pushovers. However, if they take an honest look at themselves, they'll find out that even those flamboyant emotions hide their true feelings. No matter what your strategy for survival has been, take a good look at it. It was created a long time ago by someone who was little, immature, and had few resources at their disposal. It was created by your child-self.

Honor your true feelings by giving them a safe space to be expressed. In choosing the right person to share your feelings, ask yourself: *Can I trust this person to understand what I feel without giving me unsolicited advice? Can I trust this person not to take what I say personally and get hurt by my words?*

Many of my clients love to share all their emotions with their partners and get frustrated if they don't get the reaction they want. A partner cannot fulfill all of your needs, and expecting them to is asking the impossible. Search for a trusted friend, a counselor, or a spiritual guide to share some of your feelings. Remember, you also have pen and paper and your Higher Power, who will always be there to listen.

As you are beginning to understand and work on your right to be here—for you have chosen to come into this world—and your right to have the birthing experience you desire—the same or different from your cultural or familial indoctrination—you begin to understand how your feelings play a big part in your well-being. When we feel good about ourselves and our ability to make the right choices, even if they differ from the norm, we can focus on what it is we really want.

YOUR RIGHT TO WANT

It is time to have clear intentions. Where you are going to have the baby, who you want to be present at the birth, and who you want to have as a care provider are all pivotal questions that need to be decided as you embark on a journey toward a painless childbirth.

WHERE ARE YOU GOING TO HAVE THE BABY, AND WHO WILL BE YOUR CARE PROVIDER?

Here are some questions to ask a care provider and the representative of the facility in which you decide to have your baby.[16]

1. *How do you feel about a natural childbirth?* Pay attention to your care provider's answers. You are looking for someone who respects your desires; someone who is

willing to spend time with you and honor your decisions.

2. *How would you feel if we wanted to work with a doula?* Whether you decide to hire a doula or not, this question will reveal your care provider's willingness to support your desire for a natural birth.

3. *Can you help us find childbirth classes and breastfeeding classes?* A care provider who has a list of resources is one who cares deeply for your preparation. It is important to have access to pre- and post-natal support, such as lactation consultants, childbirth education classes, pediatricians, support groups for breastfeeding mothers, etc.

4. *How many of your clients give birth without the use of pain medications? How do you feel about working with these women?* A caring provider will want you to experience the kind of birth you want, and will be happy to utilize the least amount of medical interventions necessary.

5. *How many days past my EDD (estimated due date) are you comfortable waiting for my labor to begin?* Make sure your desires are very clear about how long you would like to wait before being medically induced. Gestation can usually go up to two weeks after the due date with safe weekly or bi-weekly fetal monitoring.

6. *What is the routine procedure once a laboring woman enters your facility?* Make sure that your chosen birth setting encourages different methods for a natural labor and delivery, such as allowing a woman to move around and assume different positions during labor and delivery. Also, make sure that you will be able to hold the baby and breastfeed immediately following the birth and that the hospital will allow your baby to stay with you after the delivery in your postpartum room.

7. *How many of your clients are induced to start labor? How many clients in the last month had to be induced? How*

many women who didn't plan for Cesarean birth ended up with one, and what were the reasons? Ask for specific numbers.

8. *Aside from offering drugs, what do you suggest I do to stay comfortable during labor?* People who care for you should know how to help you cope with labor using alternative comfort measures. You may want to choose a provider who will not try to convince you that drugs are the only way to manage labor. All drugs affect the baby in some way. As much as we do not want to focus on what can go wrong, it is important to be prepared. Knowing the facility's continuum of pain management techniques is important.

9. *What if the baby is born early or has special problems?* Will the mother and family members be allowed to touch, hold, breastfeed, and care for the baby as much as possible even if the baby is in an incubator? What about kangaroo care?[17]

10. *Does this hospital circumcise, vaccinate, or perform other interventions to the babies as a routine procedure? What are those procedures?* Medical research shows there is no need to circumcise baby boys. Circumcision hurts and removes a very sensitive piece of anatomy placed there for its own divine reason. If you are going to go through with this procedure, please be sure to ask if one of the parents can be present and comfort the child during it, and if you can breastfeed immediately following the procedure. Vaccinations should be thoroughly discussed with your pediatrician. No vaccinations are needed at birth.

11. *What if I want to deliver my child on all fours?* This question is designed to see how far away from standard hospital procedures your care provider is willing to go. You may not want to end up on your hands and knees, but

what you are looking for is a response similar to this: "As long as you can efficiently push your baby out, I don't care which position you choose to do it in."

IF YOU ARE INTERVIEWING A MIDWIFE, USE THESE QUESTIONS:

1. *Do you have a medical doctor that backs you up?* As much as we don't want to focus on what can go wrong, we also want to work with someone who, in the event of a transport to the hospital, will be supported by a doctor that will understand your desire for a homebirth and will not make you feel bad or ashamed for your decision.

2. *Aside from you, who else will be present at the homebirth?* Most midwives work with at least one assistant, and many have a few training midwives to assist them. Make sure you feel comfortable having many people around. For some of us, the more the merrier, but for some, two other women are just plenty. Advocate for what feels right to you.

3. *How long have you been a midwife? How many hospital transports have you had and why?* These are routine questions to help you assess the extent of your midwife's experience and her level of self-confidence. You'll also find out what the midwife considers a dangerous birth. By talking to more than one midwife, you'll be able to see the different approaches to medical emergencies. Some midwives are conservative, and some have a more lax approach. You want to choose the one that fits with your personality. Trust your gut feelings, ask yourself how comfortable you feel around this person, not just how knowledgeable you think she is.

4. *If the baby is breech, will you perform a version yourself or will you have a doctor do it? How long before the due date*

will you do it? Unfortunately, most midwives and doctors will no longer deliver a breech baby (a baby that is not in a head-down position) vaginally. A version is a manual maneuver that attempts to turn the baby around. There is a great deal of debate over when it should be done. Most doctors will not perform one before the thirty-eighth week of gestation, as it is possible for the mother to go into labor after such a maneuver. Yet some believe that having one done so late is often unsuccessful, because the baby is already so big, giving it little room to turn around. It is important to find someone who will discuss her knowledge with you and will allow you to make your own decision.[18]

5. *How many births do you have a month, and do you have a backup?* Of course, no one can be available twenty-four hours a day, seven days a week. Look for a midwife who has a backup, and who can guarantee that you will have support for the homebirth you desire.

6. *When do you come to the house?* Some midwives will come at the last minute and will give you little support during the whole labor. There is nothing wrong with that, but you might want a doula to come early and help you manage the contractions. Some midwives will come and check on you, then leave and come back. Make sure you understand what your midwife does and ask for references.

7. *What birth preparation classes do you offer?* Some midwives offer birth preparation classes included in their packages, and some don't. Find out if they can refer you to classes to get prepared. Doulas will usually help you in this department as well.

It's OK to bring these questions with you to your first visit. Care providers respect people who are informed.

Empower yourself to find the provider you really want. It is important to be jovial, pleasant, and not confrontational. Make sure that your care provider does not feel you will challenge him or her every step of the way. Tell them that you are asking a lot of questions ahead of time so that you may relax in your pregnancy knowing that you will be supported in your desire for a safe, natural, and drug-free birth. Share all these questions with your partner and ask if there is anything important they want to add. Again, trust that you have a right to know who the provider is and what is their standard of practice. As a part of your sacred journey, think of your care provider as the navigator and yourself as the captain.

Many of my clients feel afraid the doctor will get offended if they ask for references or ask too many questions. Yet they have no problem interviewing people and checking references when hiring anyone for the firm they work for or when interviewing a doula, a nanny, or even a housekeeper. In fact, we consider it common sense to put in this due diligence. Why is it, then, that when we hire someone who will have our well-being in his/her hands, we abdicate our right to know? For the most part, it is due to a cultural fallacy. At times, we feel so beneath the doctors that we think asking these questions is stepping beyond our boundaries. Today, we are learning to do things differently; we are learning to use our common sense instead of just relying on what our culture believes is adequate. As long as there is compassion, gentleness, respect, and love, all questions are acceptable. After all, it is your body, your baby, and your birth.

HOMEBIRTH, HOSPITAL BIRTH, BIRTHING CENTER?

Before we address the best place for you to have your baby, I would like to appeal to your own intuition. These days, many women decide to have a child later in life. If this is the case for you, you might be told that you could be (or are) in the high-risk category. I personally don't believe age in and of itself makes a difference; a more comprehensive assessment of your medical history is more informative than the number of your years and a bunch of statistics. In Spain, a sixty-seven-year-old woman recently gave birth to healthy twins. This story, and others like it, demonstrates that age is relative. Your attitude and self-confidence are also a big part of the equation. If you feel strongly one way or another, please have enough information and seek several professional opinions before you abdicate and allow yourself to be labeled high-risk. Giving birth is one of the most important events in the life of a human being.

Some women spend thousands of dollars on their wedding dresses, yet when they find out how much it costs to have a baby at home, and that their insurance will not cover it, they feel they cannot justify the money. I even hear such arguments for the cost of a doula, which is a lot lower. Consider how important the birth is to your child for the rest of his life. Think of how you will feel about yourself, empowered to have the kind of birthing experience you truly desire. Having a successful birth has been shown to make a substantial difference in the postpartum stage. A confident mother takes care of her child better than one who has relinquished her powers to any other authority figure. Go inside and ask your child how he or she would like to come into this world.

HOMEBIRTH

I had two homebirths and am admittedly partial to them. It was very important for me to know that all the people who were going to be around me and my child at home would not only be there to care for us, but that they deeply loved us. Knowing that my child would never be handled by an over-tired, underpaid, and overworked nurse also made me feel better. Knowing that the lights could be lowered, the atmosphere could be gentler, and the transition more natural made me stand by my decision. Yet I respect anyone who feels more confident at the hospital, and I do not challenge her choice. I also believe that you can bring a little home into any institution, for indeed, home is where the heart is. I have observed that when we live in a state of unconditional love and compassion for ourselves and others, people are transformed by our love.

In an article entitled "Home Births Safe for Most,"[19] researchers compared the outcomes of 862 planned home births attended by midwives with those of planned hospital births attended by either midwives (571) or physicians (743) during the years 1998 and 1999. The results of the study showed that women who gave birth at home attended by a midwife had fewer procedures during labor compared with women who gave birth in a hospital attended by a physician.

Women who give birth at home usually have a healthy, normal birth. Drugs are not an option, and it is amazing how women step up to the challenge and have a wonderful, unmedicated birth. Most emergencies are handled successfully with no-risk, low-tech strategies and instrumentation. For thousands of years, women of all ages have given birth at home and have had perfectly healthy children.

Of course, there are precautions to be taken in the home-birth process. The first and foremost is that your caregiver is well trained and competent. It is also important that a hospital is not more than approximately thirty minutes from your home.

At home, you can enlist all the support you need to achieve a natural childbirth. You can use a water tub, you can have your music, your comforts, your family and friends. At home, you can eat and drink as much as you wish, you are surrounded by familiar images, and you know where and how to calm yourself. Once you give birth, you will not need to go anywhere. If there are other children, they can participate, or they can simply wake up to their new brother or sister without much of a shock. At home, your baby will snuggle up with you and your partner from the very first night (more on co-sleeping in the tenth chapter) and the three of you will bond divinely. It will be up to you to prepare your sacred space to birth your baby, and you will feel empowered and supported by your ancestry.

BIRTHING CENTERS

Unfortunately, the number of birthing centers available in the United States is decreasing. Nevertheless, if one is available to you, a birthing center is certainly a good alternative to a hospital. Birthing centers generally encourage the birthing woman to handle her contractions using natural methods, and the absence of drugs allows her to focus on the labor process, rather than be numb to it.

Most emergencies at birthing centers are handled on site, with low-tech equipment, and most centers are no more than thirty minutes away from the hospital. Other advantages of using a birthing center are access to a whirlpool or birthing tub, and of course the bonus of having someone else clean up. In most cases, the baby is not separated from the mother, but depending on the birthing center, you might be handled by several different people on several shifts.

A birthing center is a great choice if you feel uncomfortable with your home setting or if you live far away from medical facilities. Birthing centers have either a medical doctor on staff or guaranteed medical backup and are well equipped for minor emergencies (just like midwives). Birthing centers also provide a sense of legitimacy for family and partners who are worried about a homebirth.

Hospital Births

As soon as you enter the hospital in labor, you are offered a wheelchair. In an instant, it seems as if you are transformed from a beautiful laboring mother, with nothing wrong but the onset of the natural waves of labor, to an incapacitated patient who needs to be evaluated, hooked up to machines, and automatically medicated. Later in this book, we will address how to handle arriving at the hospital. For now, let's simply weigh the pros and cons of the hospital as a birth setting. In a hospital, a nurse will care for you, but she will leave at the end of her shift (usually a twelve hour shift from 7 a.m. to 7 p.m. and vice versa), at which time a new nurse will take over. She will likely be in telephone contact with the doctor, who will choose the course of action based on her evaluation, not on your desires. In addition to taking care of you, a nurse will be responsible for up to three or four other laboring women. Her obligation to different patients limits her abilities in personal and emotional care, two factors that are so important to the comfort of an expectant mother. As much as most nurses are giving, kind, and experienced people, many are highly overworked and overburdened with patients and doctors' orders.

If choosing a hospital birth, I appeal to you to make a connection with your nurse right away. Making him or her an ally from the start can make your birthing experience easier. However, if the chemistry is simply not there, it is a good idea to ask your partner to get in touch with the head nurse and ask to be assigned to another nurse. It is your right to have a supportive nurse by your side.

In the hospital, the doctor usually arrives at the last pushing phase to deliver the child. On average, this is thirty minutes to two hours before the baby is out. Indeed, if something were to go terribly wrong, the hospital is the best place to be. However, be aware that the proximity of all the high-tech equipment can result in its overuse. The fact that drugs are readily available and are constantly offered makes this place one where you will have to use a lot more willpower to stay the course for a natural childbirth.

Remember, hospitals are businesses, and they run accordingly. The primary goal of an efficient business is to process you as expediently as possible, so as to have the room/bed open for the next patient. Thus, there is often an underlying tendency to not allow, and even to discourage, the wait for the natural course of birth to happen. If you do not progress according to a standard timeline, you might be offered Pitocin, a synthetic hormone that increases or starts contractions, often offered to speed up or kick start your labor.

Many hospitals these days are trying to create a gentler environment with homelike birthing rooms. However, at the hospital, you may feel really alone unless you bring someone aside from your partner with you, like a doula, friend, or birth coach.

No matter what your logic tells you, your unconscious mind will probably be on alert, because the hospital environment is often associated with negative past experiences. Until now, it is likely that you have gone to the hospital only if there was something wrong. Your body, mind, and spirit will remember these past experiences and you'll have to work hard to calm them down. I have had clients who literally used the hospital for only one to two hours to birth their babies, after having labored at home for the greatest part of their labor.

Once you have decided where and with whom you are going to have your child, you need to find out if there is anything inside yourself that needs healing. You must heal your mind, soul, and body as you prepare for this new phase in your life. This brings us to the importance of visiting your own birth. Here's how one woman did it.

Julie's Story

Julie feared she couldn't take care of her newborn daughter, Lisa. She had constant nightmares and was unable to sleep well. Recognizing that these might be the beginning symptoms of postpartum depression, Julie went to a therapist who suggested she have some hypnotherapy sessions.

In her first e-mail to me, she wrote: "I can't concentrate. I need help with the anxiety I've been experiencing. There are other issues, but the bottom line is that I want to be a good mother to my daughter and a good partner to my husband, and I can't do this until I find a sense of peace and balance within myself." In our first meeting, we went through a step-by-step regression to revisit her own birth.

Julie's Mom's Story

Julie's mom, a seventeen-year-old girl named Tate, hid her pregnancy for a very long time because she felt ashamed and scared. Tate's parents wanted her to give her child up for adoption. They had other plans for her. They wanted her to finish school, go to college, get married, and then have children. Throughout her pregnancy, Tate fought for her right to have her baby, but she constantly felt that her battle was a losing one. Even her boyfriend, who was initially on her side, abandoned her. Tate felt completely alone. Sad, depressed, and tired of all the fighting, Tate resigned to her parents' desires and entered a house for troubled girls. For a short period, Tate felt happier. She spent her time listening to music and began talking to her unborn child. But the peace evaporated when Tate learned that the shelter specialized in adoption. She ran away and hid at her sister's house. She gave birth in a lot of pain, and as a young mother, she was constantly in and out of trouble. Tate died when Julie was only seventeen years old, and Julie was adopted by her grandparents.

Julie Recalls Her Feelings Inside the Womb

Julie enters a deep state of hypnosis. Her first memories are of her spirit feeling fear and sadness. She wants to be born to her mom and is happy to leave the place her spirit inhabited before conception. When Julie is a four-week-old embryo, she begins to feel her mother's emotions: nervous, scared, isolated, and alone. By the third month she hears herself scream, "No more secrets, mom!" Julie wants her mom to be happy, but she also feels impatient.

Julie hears the family fights. She hears her mom standing up for herself and for her right to want this child. She feels like screaming, "Give them hell, Mom! It's your right to have me!"

In the third trimester, while Tate is at the house for troubled girls, Julie remembers sleeping a lot. She sees the womb as a dark and quiet place. She feels a strong connection with her mother and falls in love with her.

Empowered by that love, Julie declares, "Don't worry, Mom, I will take care of you." *This is a solid pact that will color most of Julie's childhood.*

Of her actual birth, all Julie remembers is her mother's pain. As a newborn, she remembers being quiet, sleeping a lot, and not daring to cry, even when she is in her crib alone. When her mom picks her up, Julie looks into her mother's eyes and tries to convey the message, "Don't worry, Mom, I am here, I'll help." As she grows up,

Julie tries to be a good girl. She never asks for what she wants, figuring this will make her mom's life easier. Yet her mom is never happy, always worried, and hardly ever around. Julie feels she has failed. When her mother dies, Julie is just seventeen years old. She feels lost—she was unable to take care of her mom. Now that she lives with her grandparents, she resigns and declares, "I will never get what I want." *This is the second pact, which will influence most of Julie's adult life.*

We spent several more sessions on her early years. Julie brought her adult-self each time she went back into her memory and began re-parenting herself and even caring for her mother, which ultimately fulfilled her first promise. She began working on her right to be here in this world, her right to have a happy family, and her right to her feelings: wanting serenity and freedom from her past. Her affirmation was: "I am loving, lovable, and loved. All I want is within my reach. I am capable of being a good person to myself, a good mother to my daughter, and a good partner to my husband."

After a few months, Julie felt much better, even in the midst of the family crisis that arose when her aunt died suddenly. She reported she was amazed at how she could handle her sadness with renewed strength. By remembering the solemn pacts we have made in our early childhood, we can dispel their influence in our lives. Awareness is the first step toward transformation. The past is not carved in stone; by changing our memories we can heal it. Such an understanding will bring you closer to a painless childbirth.

HEALING YOUR WOMB

Whether a pregnancy is planned or simply happens, we are all part of a bigger design, nature's design. In light of the need to let go of all past experiences that could color the outcome of this birth, we need to look at and heal events that are directly related to past births, terminations, miscarriages, and deaths. If this is not your first pregnancy, you may want to spend time healing the strong feelings associated with your last experience.

Maybe your first delivery was not what you wanted. Some of you had to have a Cesarean birth and are unhappy with that. Others had many medical interventions that left you and/or your child debilitated or depressed. Maybe you felt you had no control during the birth process and are angry as a result. Perhaps you have pushed these feelings down, but now fear and resentment well up, and you seem to be unable to forget what happened.

Some of you carried a child for a while and you lost him/her unexpectedly in a miscarriage. Or perhaps you had to have a termination. Or, worse yet, you carried a child full term, but he or she did not live.

Just because something happened in the past does not mean it will repeat itself. When it comes to healing a Cesarean birth you are not happy about, I want you to consider that despite what many doctors say—"Once a Cesarean, always a Cesarean"—you do have a choice and can have a vaginal birth (also called VBAC—Vaginal Birth After Cesarean). There is a lot to know about VBACs, and I encourage you to research your options. Right now, let's focus on healing the wounds from any of these past experiences.

I have spoken to women who lost their child at full term and were very angry at God. I understand that reaction. I would like to take a moment to talk to those women now.

I know that the system does not recognize your baby, that you have struggled to get a birth certificate, not just a death certificate. You have wondered whether you can be considered a mom, since you could not bring the baby home. I would like to extend a heartfelt hug to you and acknowledge your baby, whether he/she was three gestational weeks old or lived for nine months or a few years on this earth. You were blessed by their presence. You carried them and enjoyed their Divine expression with pride and joy. You are indeed a parent. Don't let anyone tell you differently. Such children never leave you. They have a sacred place in your heart. If this current pregnancy has come after you've lost a baby, I suspect that your only focus might be to bring a baby home, no matter what the pain during labor is, no matter if you'll give birth naturally or not. I hear you, I see you, I agree with you, and I want you to know that I recognize that the death of your baby is a tragedy and that the impact of that loss was enormous on the lives of your entire family. As terrible as the outcome was, that child was important not only to your family, but to the entire universe. We are all like pebbles thrown into the water. No matter how big or small, we all create concentric waves that will eventually touch every shore the water touches. Thus, each of us has an impact on everything and everyone. His presence was not in vain; her life, however brief, is significant.

For all women who have lost a baby or who have had to terminate a pregnancy, I encourage you to deal with it early on in your new pregnancy. I encourage you to talk about it with a therapist, and/or join support groups.

Regardless of what has happened in the past, I strongly suggest using writing as part of your own healing process. I have found that writing a series of letters is very useful. Write one letter to each of those people you are still mad at because of what happened. Definitely write a letter to God, your doctor, yourself, your baby, and to anyone else you think should hear what you have to say. Write what happened. You can simply say, "I am writing to tell you about the miscarriage I had (or the angel I didn't bring home)," and switch to what you want to tell them. If you choose to, you can write out every little detail of what happened. Go ahead and allow all of your feelings to surface. Get angry if you need to. Use insults, get sad, and let it all come out. You will not send these letters! They are meant for your eyes only.

It's important to stay focused on the process. Indeed, allow your feelings to surface freely, but try to experience them as a witness without falling into the abyss. Bring yourself back to the here and now so that you can use this exercise to work through what happened, without getting stuck in it.

Next, write what you would like to happen this time, this birth, and ask every recipient for their support. Be specific as to how you would like to be supported this time (this you will definitely use later on as you express your desires to your partner, your doctor or midwife, and all the people on your list). Make a commitment to yourself that you will take charge of your pregnancy and that, no matter what, you will establish a good relationship with your child in the womb. Cherish every minute of this pregnancy, trying not to color this new event with fear and trepidation from what happened in the past.

Recognize that nothing in life is permanent. Do this so that this child may rejoice in your womb and not swim in terrorized waters, so that you can be replenished with love and trust from within. This is a very emotional exercise, but things left unsaid or unfelt do linger in our consciousness. Once they are out in the open, healing can begin.

There will be no need to fight with those you hold responsible. The purpose of this exercise is to forgive your doctor, your partner, God, and yourself. Resentment lingers and festers, and nothing good ever comes from it. An old adage says, "Resentment is like taking poison and waiting for the other person to die." Tell the baby you lost that you've reserved a special place in your heart for them. Tell them that you love and accept them.

If you are angry because you wanted a natural childbirth and ended up with a different birthing experience, tell yourself that the birth you had was perfect as it was, for it taught you to search out a way to do things differently this time. After this writing, you will feel lighter and you will be able to tackle this birth with renewed intentions.

Be gentle and mother yourself. Rejoice that you have already done so much good work in preparing yourself for the birthing experience you have a right to want.

Be Grateful

What are you thankful for? Take inventory of all your blessings. Yes, all of them. Add one new item daily. Consider the following: family, friends, faith, health, the child that is growing inside you, the morning dew, the sunset, fresh air, and all that is awesome in the universe. We each have 1,440 minutes in every day. How would your life be different if you spent just fifteen of those minutes each day being grateful for what you have? Focus your attention on those things that show how fortunate you are. After a few days, you will discover that this exercise is truly life-changing.

MONTH

3

the right to act

*I am confident in my actions. I have an innate ability to discern
what is right for my pregnancy and my child. I am here to inspire
my unborn baby to trust herself and to see her actions as inspired
by her Higher Self. I believe that a painless birth is the reality my
baby and I will experience together. We will intuitively know how
to proceed each step of the way, inspiring my baby to trust her
own actions. I offer my life over to the care of my Higher Power,
and I am thankful for the gifts I receive. Knowing that all my
needs are met, I simply let them go. And so it is. Amen.*

YOUR BABY NOW

Your baby is now three to four inches long, crown to rump, and weighs about an ounce—the equivalent of about half of a banana. Its unique fingerprints are already in place. When you poke your stomach gently, he feels it and will start rooting, acting as if he's searching for a nipple. He has the ability to swallow, absorb, and discharge fluids. His hands are now complete and growing fingernails. Even tooth buds are emerging. Your baby's face now has a distinctly human appearance.

THE THIRD CHAKRA

The third chakra relates to our right to act. It is located in the lower belly. It is the seat of one's personal power. It directly affects our ability to project our will into manifestation. In this chakra, we focus on personal power and we explore our right to take action. Your baby begins to move and respond to stimuli at around ten weeks of life in the womb. Expressions of interest and of protest against uncomfortable experiences have been observed during ultrasound tests.[20] Something as simple as a mother's laugh or cough will provoke an action by the fetus. Research[21] has shown that during amniocentesis,[22] the baby reacts aggressively to the needle, suggesting self-protection, self-assertion, and expressions of fear and anger. The baby is learning its right to take action within its own environment. This confirms the importance of becoming conscious of your daily actions, rather than defaulting into unconscious behavior.

THE RIGHT TO ACT

Nothing happens unless you make it happen. If you want something to change, you must act. An excellent definition of insanity is, "doing the same thing over and over again, expecting different results." Such a path never provides happiness, harmony, prosperity, success, peace, or balance. You must do something different if you want to see different results.

Become mindful of your daily routines, starting with your morning ritual. Every morning, you wake up and go through a ritual to take care of your body. You start by going to the bathroom. Then, you may go into the kitchen and drink coffee or tea, then back to the bathroom to get ready. You spend some time on your face, maybe applying makeup, or brushing and styling your hair. You carefully choose your clothes and eventually leave the house, securely closing the door behind you. You think you have taken care of everything, but you haven't taken a minute to step out of your routine and compose yourself. It takes only five precious minutes to set our intentions for the day and to connect our mind and our soul to our Higher Self. Those five minutes are your most important ones. They determine the course of your actions. Practice closing your eyes for five minutes before you even get up from bed and either think of all the things you are grateful for, or repeat a simple affirmation: *Today I feel unstoppable, life is so good. I feel good, I feel great.*

In order to bring consciousness to your actions you must first know what they are. Make a list of the rituals you perform each day and begin to slowly make some changes. Modify the actions you take habitually and become conscious of your routine. Try this simple exercise: if you always drive to work via the same route, change it. By paying attention to the road, you will learn to stay in the here and now. If you usually wear dark clothes, begin adding color to your wardrobe. This way you will awaken your child-self. If you are talkative, be quiet and listen. This will teach you to pay attention to the people around you. If you are the reserved type, start making small conversation with strangers at the supermarket or at the post office. Making these small changes might not feel comfortable at first, but sometimes just doing things differently will cast new light onto situations, allowing a different aspect of yourself to come to life.

NEGATIVE ACTIONS AND THEIR REWARDS

Sometimes we create negative actions for the rewards they bring. If you've heard yourself say, "That's just the way I am. I can't help it," realize that this statement is a declaration of how unwilling you are to change. If you are the type of person who often says, "Nothing really good happens to me," or "I never get what I want," you are probably right. When you truly believe those statements and act accordingly, you make them come true because what we focus on expands. Here's a story that illustrates this concept.

Actions Follow Our Belifs

I once had a boyfriend who would say, "I always seem to be in some kind of trouble." He would laugh about his car blowing up, or having to go to the emergency room on Thanksgiving day, or having to go to court because a mechanic sold him a lemon. He thought he had a great sense of humor because he was able to laugh at these adversities, yet his continual refrain, "Something awful always happens to me," actually reinforced this reality. All his actions and efforts were centered on fixing things or getting others to help him out of trouble, which only attracted more bad things. Since his troubles always took center stage, it was impossible for his friends to ask *him* for help.

One day, I proposed that he find the one positive reward in all of his negative drama. "Well," he said, "one thing I can say is that I have great friends who come and help me anytime I need them." He admitted that he measured his friends' loyalty by how much they were willing to do for him in an emergency. The more they were ready to help him, the more he felt loved. He believed that absent of drama and crisis, he would not have any true friends.

I sent him a note with this affirmation: "The more friends I have, the less drama comes to my life, and the more I can be of service and feel worthy." I also suggested that he switch things around for two weeks and only telephone his friends to learn how they were doing, and not dwell on his circumstances, no matter what was going on in his life.

Here's what he told me after the two-week experiment: "The most amazing thing I learned was that I had spent so little time listening to other people's lives that I didn't even know some of them had really serious problems. But even more incredible is that by talking to them about their lives, my dramas just became smaller. By no means has my life become all smooth sailing, but now as soon as something happens to me, I pick up the phone and turn my attention to what I can do for a friend, and I feel better. The feeling of shame I felt before, every time I thought about how I could ask a friend to do one more thing for me, is gone. I hate to say it, but it's working."

To turn your destiny around, you must take action and change. Start by asking yourself what recurring phrases you use to describe yourself, your life, and your future birthing experience. Maybe you've heard yourself saying things like:

- "I want to have a natural, painless childbirth with no medical interventions, but I am chicken when it comes to pain."
- "I am not lucky. What I want never really happens."

- "I don't even want to think about how the birth will be, or else I'll jinx it."

Let's start by making a list of the "rewards" you receive when you share those statements with others. For example:

- When I say those things, my partner puts his arms around me and tells me everything will be OK.
- I feel humble. I avoid tempting fate when I say, "I am not lucky."
- If I expect the worst, I will be prepared should it come to pass.
- I am superstitious. If I wish for the best, I will only get its opposite. I feel safer not thinking about it.

Take note of how you describe who you are and what your expectations are. Initially, you may become frustrated by how many times you catch yourself repeating your negative spiel. Bear in mind that the act of catching yourself makes you more attentive and brings you closer to changing your habits and creating a new you.

A state of serenity, success, and happiness is the single most important factor for the successful outcome of your birth. Strip away your fears and take action toward a new way of thinking and feeling, one small step at a time.

POSITIVE ACTIONS

Another important action to take in manifesting your desired birthing experience, is to write, in detail, the story of your labor and delivery as you desire and intend it to be. Here's a sample script from one of my clients.

Script by Margaret

Early labor comes on gently at night. I awaken with contractions and I am excited. I wake my husband up and tell him I think this is it. He smiles and helps me go back to sleep with a soothing massage and a cup of tea. We tell our baby to prepare for the long day ahead and to go to sleep while I sing him a lullaby. Listening to a meditation tape helps me manage the waves and I go back to sleep for a few hours. In the morning, we go to my favorite breakfast place for chocolate chip pancakes. Every once in a while, I have to stop to manage a contraction. They are mild and it is easy to do. I feel so happy and a little apprehensive, so I discuss it with John. He tells me he is confident I can do it and allows me to feel my feelings. We leave the restaurant and go to the beach for a walk. The morning air is crisp and the colors are beautiful. I can hear the roaring of the waves and I take deep breaths of fresh air. When the contractions come, I put my arms around John and we slow dance. I feel so proud and lucky to have such a wonderful companion with me. John is such a trouper. I know he is scared, but he has great self-control and he is my rock. We return home and I get into the tub, as John calls the midwife and my doula. When it's time to push the baby out, I simply stay in the tub and our child peeks his head out effortlessly. I reach for him and place him on my bosom. I look at him in awe—he is mine; I can't believe it!

Details are important, but even more are the feelings you experience when you read your story. You are setting your intentions and taking action toward the goal of a natural and painless childbirth.

Once this vision is written, read it to yourself. Some of my clients have recorded themselves reading their stories and listen to them on their iPods as they go for their daily walk. Remember, once it is written, you can always modify it, embellish it, and rewrite it.

If you prefer, you can draw or paint the perfect birthing experience. Be sure to use color to show the atmosphere that will surround you, draw the people that will be there, and infuse the canvas with your feelings. Hang it up somewhere in your bedroom and as you look at it, feel the joy and ease of your upcoming birth.

OUR ACTIONS ARE BORN: WILLINGNESS IS THE KEY
A Birth Story

FEAR NOT, LITTLE FLOCK, FOR IT IS YOUR FATHER'S GOOD PLEASURE TO GIVE YOU THE KINGDOM. (LUKE 12:32)

"If there is a will, there is a wall." Once I heard this at my spiritual center, I could not get it out of my head. I was raised with the exact opposite dictum: "Where there's a will, there's a way." I'd always pushed hard to get where I wanted to go. I had a will—a strong will—and by God, I was going to find the way to get where I wanted to be.

Instead of focusing on the strength of our will, Reverend Dr. Michael Beckwith proposes that we let go of our self-will and become willing to receive what we desire instead of fighting for it. After hearing this message, I realized that even when willfulness had seemed to be working in my life, a wall indeed arose somehow, somewhere. For instance, I once tried to pressure a publisher into publishing my book. My will was strong and I engaged everyone I knew to send him e-mails, telling him to do so. The publisher initially loved the idea of my book, but once he proposed it to his staff, they rallied against it. Without even reading the proposal, the project was turned down. I'd call that a serious karmic wall!

In reviewing the births I have witnessed, and passing them through the sieve of will versus willingness, I noticed a blueprint. If I, or a client, stand firm in our will to have a certain outcome during the birth, a wall gets thrown up. Whether it comes from the nurses, doctors, or even the client's unconscious, ego begets ego and resistance is usually the outcome. On the other hand, when having formed a clear vision of the birth and having set our intentions, we enter the birth setting with love in our hearts and the willingness to be open and receptive, the outcome is a natural and painless childbirth. Shortly after learning this lesson, I had the following experience.

I worked with Mary and Jay for about two months. Among other things in our prenatal visits, I explained the pros and cons of vaginal exams performed at every doctor's visit. Serial vaginal examinations at thirty-six through thirty-nine weeks can be discouraging and have no bearing on the outcome and progress of the pregnancy. Yet, Mary would call me weekly, telling me that she had been checked again. As expected, finding out that she had not dilated and was just a little effaced was making her nervous. I urged her to ask why her doctor felt the need to check her so often. I encouraged her to convey her desire to participate in the decision-making.

Mary seemed unable to say no, or to ask for what she wanted. I noticed that *I* was getting concerned. Under hypnosis, she revealed that her major apprehension was to be unable to stand by her decision of having a drug-free birth. Despite her strong desire for a natural birth, Mary wanted to be reassured that she could have an epidural if she felt she needed one. I told her that she was in charge of her birthing experience, and that I was there to support her decision no matter what, without any judgments. I further suggested she should be free of self-judgment, regardless of what her ultimate decision was going to be. In other words, she would simply let the moment and the circumstances dictate the outcome. She needed to become willing to accept nature's plan for her, and so did I.

During another hypnotherapy session, she had a wonderful conversation with her unborn child, named after the Balinese goddess, Sinta who, with a mothering tone, told her to relax and not to worry, for the birth was going to be great. When the baby talked to her mother, the room filled with a sense of quiet and serenity. Sinta was a true goddess. She radiated self-confidence from within her mother's womb. I could tell this was going to be a very special experience.

Later in the session, Mary remembered how she had succeeded in completing a twenty-two-mile marathon. She recalled that during the run she had nearly given up several times, but somehow found the strength to move forward and finish. I suggested she harness that experience and transfer her determination from the marathon onto the birth.

Mary was ready. She had the skill and the intention, and she had enlisted her daughter's Divine power. As her doula, I had to become willing to see a perfect birth for her, despite her reluctance to set limits with the doctor.

Her contractions started in the early morning hours, five days before her due date. At 8:00 a.m., she called to tell me that the contractions were coming every twenty minutes. She was managing them and was calm. By 10:00 a.m., they had switched to every ten minutes, and she was happily listening to my self-hypnosis CD while her mom and husband were caring for her. At noon, she requested that I join her. Usually, early labor with the first baby can last a very long time, and it is better to use this time connecting with your partner, so I was a little reluctant to join them so early. But my intuition suggested I go to her. When I arrived at her house, I found Mary smiling radiantly between contractions that were frequent and strong. We decided she needed a nap, so with the help of hypnosis she rested for about an hour. We then took a walk around her neighborhood, enjoying the amazing roses in bloom. Once back home, I suggested she take a relaxing bath. By then it was around 3:00 p.m. She lay in the warm tub and rode the mounting waves of contractions beautifully; it looked like Mom and Goddess Sinta were dancing a private and peaceful dance.

During her bath, I noticed what looked like involuntary pushing. In second stage contractions, the pressure of the baby in the vagina and the pressure on the rectum can cause a mother to feel a strong need to groan, hold her breath, and bear down. This urge can be as irresistible as the urge to sneeze. Resisting it can be more difficult than simply surrendering and letting it happen.

As a result, we realized that it was time to go to the hospital. The ride took forty minutes, and I made sure Mary had a ritual—a specific position, breathing technique, and sound to use during the contractions while in the car. Usually the ride to the hospital can change the tone of the labor because at home the waves may be manageable, but a bumpy car ride can take a woman's focus away. In my experience, it is important to be prepared and have a plan during transport.

Upon checking into the hospital, the nurse casually directed us to triage, assuming that there was no urgent need to check Mary, announcing, "She doesn't have the labor face." The expression "labor face" is a common way that some hospital nurses judge labor's progress. In other words, if you are smiling and composed and this is your first baby, they may assume that you have come to the hospital too early, and as a result of their bias, you have to insist on being checked, which is exactly what I did since our nurse had disappeared. I went to the nurses' station and told the head nurse that Mary was involuntarily pushing and that someone needed to check her right away. The resident doctor came over, and as she checked for dilation, Mary's water broke in a gush. "She's nine centimeters dilated and fully effaced," declared the resident. "We should call her doctor and put her in a room."

My going to the nurses' station had raised a wall. I felt tension from the nurses who settled Mary into the room. They insisted on IV fluids and told her to stop pushing, for they feared her cervix would swell up even though she was fully effaced. They demanded she stay perfectly still as they asked a barrage of questions, and were determined she should wait for her doctor to arrive. All these procedures at this juncture seemed to ignore the needs of the woman, giving precedence to hospital regulations. No one seemed to pay attention to the fact that this baby was about to be born and that Mary needed support, not resistance. Anger was sneaking into my consciousness.

So I decided to do nothing. I closed my eyes and became willing for Mary to have the experience *she* had desired. I needed to accept the birth that she was manifesting, and fell madly in love with what was happening at that very moment. I became willing to let go of my resolve for the hospital staff to be different from who they were. I switched my attention to infuse the room with love and gratitude. Mary was stellar. She kept using, "No, thanks," as the only answer for every question posed to her, while smiling between contractions. Her husband and I bent toward Mary's belly and whispered, "Welcome, Sinta, we are ready for you whenever you are."

The resident doctor came back into the room, decreeing that Mary was probably ready to have the baby, and gave the OK to push. Mary had been pushing anyway, following her instincts and her body's desire. Her husband and I readied to help her hug, rather then push her baby out. The resident was standing by and was totally engaged. She confessed this was the first drug-free birth she had witnessed. Between contractions, and under the influence of hypnosis, Mary was easily going limp and loose, even nodding off to the surprise of all those present.

Word had spread through the hospital: a woman was

resting between contractions. She looked like she was sleeping! This was obviously something to be seen. At one point in the room, there were three resident doctors, three nurses, and three onlookers watching from the doorway.

Mary was sipping water and as the baby's head peeked in and out, I would exclaim, "Look how wonderful your baby is! She is coming out so naturally, unassisted by anyone! Look how wonderfully your perineum is stretching!" This running commentary helped to fend off doctors' meddling hands, so eager to willfully "help the baby out." Within forty minutes the baby was born. Total time in the hospital: one hour and forty minutes.

Surprisingly, and contrary to this hospital's procedure, the baby was never taken away from Mary and never placed under the warmer. Nor was the baby bathed or measured right away. It seemed that without requesting it, hospital rules were easily changed through witnessing such an amazing birth. Mary's willingness, her acceptance, her calm, and her love changed everything. I learned so much from her and from the little goddess, Sinta.

I understand now that if there is a will, if the ego is engaged, walls do come up. It is willingness we are after, the willingness to pour love into every situation, and then accept and welcome the perfection that comes our way. With this state of mind, the universe always responds. All desires are met and another painless childbirth occurs!

OTHER PEOPLE'S RIGHT TO ACT

Other people's habits can be very frustrating, especially the people we live with. Now that you are pregnant, things that didn't bother you in the past may become really annoying. You are learning to pay attention to your words, intentions, and actions, yet conflicts seem to sneak their way into your life no matter how hard you try. When you find yourself in an argument, apparently caused by other people's actions, pay attention to what you say:

- "I have told you a thousand times not to drop your dirty clothes on the floor."
- "How many times do I have to ask you to please put the toilet seat back down after you go to the bathroom?"
- "You promised before we got a dog that you would feed him and walk him, and you never do it. This is the hundredth time I've asked you, and you still don't listen."

If these sentences are familiar, or closely resemble something you have found yourself repeating over and over again getting no results, you need to look at your approach. Try modifying the way you ask for what you want. Here are some alternative ways of engaging cooperation:

- Describe the problem: "Your clothes are on the floor." Or give information: "It really helps when you pick up your clothes off the floor." Write a note and post it: "I don't like to be on the floor, please pick me up. —(signed) *Your dirty clothes*."
- Talk about your feelings: "It bothers me when the toilet seat is up, and I risk falling into the bowl."
- The fewer words, the better: "Honey, the dog."

When we take the anger and frustration out of our communication, we can achieve what we are after. This is a time to let go of your need to control how things are done by others. You are learning how to accept others' behaviors with unconditional love and compassion. As a mother, you need to practice this. Once the baby comes, and especially in the first few weeks of his life, you will have little control over your surroundings and your life.

Trust that the universe will take care of everything, including the small details. All you have to do is take care of yourself and the child in your belly.

ACTING OUT WITH FOOD

The third chakra sits between our navel and sternum, in close relation to our stomach. Just because you are pregnant doesn't mean that you should be literally eating for two. Many women, although not all, have an increased appetite once pregnant. It is OK to increase the amount you eat, as long as you are eating healthy and well-balanced meals. If your pregnancy happens around the holidays, remember that being pregnant is not giving you an automatic green light to eat all the fats or sweets you can put your hands on. Don't get me wrong. Do enjoy a large piece of pie, just don't substitute empty-calorie food for the needed proteins, vegetables, and grains.

Your water intake is important. The recommended amount is at least two quarts or eight to ten glasses, every day. Pregnant women get dehydrated easily, which can cause complications. If you don't like plain water, add juice to your water. Make sure it is 100 percent fruit juice. Or add a squeeze of fresh lemon or orange. Avoid sodas, as they are loaded with sugar and often caffeine. Electrolyte drinks are fine in moderation. They contain high amounts of sodium and potassium. One of the best drinks to prevent dehydration is coconut water.

It is thought that food cravings during pregnancy represent a way for women to get the extra nutrients their bodies need. Mother Nature, in her perfection, makes sure we provide our growing child with exactly the nutrients he needs. Many women crave meat and a particular vegetable or salad. If you're hankering for ice cream all the time, it may mean your baby is asking for more fat in your diet, or more calcium and protein. Don't let cravings for high-fat foods or sweets get out of hand.

Pregnant women generally don't need to change the amount of salt in their diet. Ask your care provider and generally stay away from high-salt foods like chips and canned goods, and don't add salt when you cook. Envision your baby eating exactly what you put in your mouth. Give her plenty of fresh fruits and vegetables, and talk to her as you do this, "My love, how would you like a juicy, fresh peach?"

THE ART OF INACTION: BED REST

About 25 percent of women are put on bed rest at some point in their pregnancy. Bed rest has been prescribed for various pregnancy complications, including risk of preterm labor, concern that the baby isn't growing properly, intrauterine growth restriction, or if the mother has placenta previa (the placenta is lying unusually low in the uterus, next to or covering the cervix). Also, the mother may be put on bed rest if she has mild gestational hypertension or preeclampsia.

There are not many conclusive studies that prove bed rest is the best solution for any or all of these symptoms. More research is needed. In the meantime, experts disagree about when and how to prescribe bed rest. Many say that until there's good evidence to the contrary, bed rest is worth it. Others disagree, stating that bed rest itself can have negative effects, and that women should not be subjected to it until we know that it does more good than harm. These caregivers tend to believe that the use of complete bed rest should be curtailed, and that some women would be better off just taking it easy, restricting their activity level, cutting back on work, avoiding heavy lifting or prolonged standing, and resting for a few hours each day.

If you have been put on bed rest, it can get pretty unnerving and discouraging, and you are going to need the tools in this book more than ever. Aside from the obvious psychological downfalls of bed rest, which include restlessness, boredom, and even depression, there is financial hardship, especially if your income is important in your family budget. Effects may also include the physical malaise of not moving, insomnia, changes in your metabolism, bone loss, and aches and pains. As always, everyone has an opinion. You have chosen your caregiver carefully and you trust in his or her opinion. If she has suggested bed rest, your choices are to listen and learn how to make the best of it, or to get a second opinion.

Another indication for bed rest can be an incompetent cervix. I prefer to call it an unskilled cervix, but common medical terms are "weak" or "incompetent" cervix. In this situation, the baby is at risk of being born prematurely because the cervix shortens or opens too early. In order to prevent early changes in a woman's cervix, a cerclage is used, thus preventing premature labor. The treatment consists of a stitch being inserted into and around the cervix early in the pregnancy, usually between weeks twelve and fourteen. The stitch is removed toward the end of the pregnancy when the greatest risk of miscarriage has passed. About 1 percent of pregnant women have a shortened cervix. With a cerclage in place, some practitioners may place certain restrictions on sexual penetration and other activities, but you don't have to stop kissing, hugging, and fondling. Usually, aerobic exercise is not permitted, although walking and isometric exercise are sometimes allowed. Cervical cerclage does not always require bed rest, or total bed rest, but the two often go hand in hand.

TEN WAYS TO COPE WITH BED REST

While most women willingly abide by the order for bed rest, for many it's an unwelcome inconvenience. There are always so many other things to do in addition to growing a baby. Yet when you consider that you will have plenty of other chances to do these things, and only one chance to complete this pregnancy, being in bed for nearly twenty-four hours a day can be managed. Take each new challenge one day at a time. Make sure you understand why you were put on bed rest. Get informed, ask questions, and request specific answers. If you can, discuss it with your doula or other birth professionals. Understanding why you are asked to do something is very important for your peace of mind. Once you feel comfortable with the decision, try to enjoy your state and see if you can fall in love with what you have to do. Here are ten ways to cope with your confinement and actually enjoy it:

1. Know exactly what you may and may not do. Be sure you understand exactly what your healthcare provider means by bed rest. You can pretty much figure that bed rest entails refraining from most activities done outside the home. However, make sure you know whether you are on total bed rest, which means sponge baths in bed and bedpans, or whether you get the luxury of bathroom privileges and an occasional walk to the kitchen. Ask if you can slowly walk up and down stairs or if you are confined to one floor. Most doctors overprescribe the degree of bed rest, realizing that most human beings do not easily adapt to such drastic changes in lifestyle, and will occasionally cheat. Ask specific questions so you don't waste hours wondering what is allowed and what is not. Can you deal with office work over the phone? How about your other children? Paint a clear picture so an overly

cautious care provider will understand what is feasible and what is asking too much for your lifestyle. Also, ask about sex and be specific: do you have to stay away from penetration and intercourse, or do you have to stay away from orgasms altogether? Depending on your condition, even an orgasm may be off limits. When you are in bed, make sure you change position often and place several pillows all around you and in between your legs.

2. Set up a comfortable nest. If you have to stay in bed, you might as well create a bed you like to stay in. Have your bed placed near or facing a window so you have fresh air and a view. Put anything you might need within arm's reach on a table next to your bed. Use a cordless phone or one with a long cord if the phone jack isn't near your bed. Keep address books, phone books, your journal, and all kinds of reading material on an adjacent table. Get lots of fun books as well as the usual instructional books. Get books on CD or tape so you don't strain yourself. Move the television or the stereo and computer into the bedroom. Buy or rent a small refrigerator for your bedside snacks. Be kind to your body.

3. Think positively. Rather than dwelling on what you're missing, think about what you are enjoying. Even if you find yourself feeling bored and depressed, these feelings will eventually subside, and you will have happy days again. Focus on what you are doing for your baby, and on the benefits of resting and relaxing. The good thing about the emotions of pregnancy is that downs are usually followed by ups. Hypnotherapy and self-hypnosis are very helpful. This is a great opportunity to work on yourself and begin a conversation with your child.

4. Realize your feelings are normal. With so much time to just sit and think, your emotions are likely to run wild.

You may worry about the baby's health and survival, fret about how your husband and kids are coping, be bored with too little to do, feel anxious about things you should be doing, and dislike feeling dependent. You may feel angry and disappointed about the course of your pregnancy. Each day in bed will bring new emotions to work through, yet continuing to focus on the goal of your pregnancy will help overcome these anxieties and keep you in bed as long as you need to stay there.

5. Seek your mate's help. This may be the first time in your life that your mate waits on you. Some women love it and others are overwhelmed with feelings of unworthiness. First of all, may I remind you that by caring for you, your partner is caring for the baby as well. Some of us are control freaks and just don't like how others do or prepare things. What a great opportunity to practice the art of letting go! Prolonged bed rest during pregnancy can bring couples together or tear them apart. He will miss your company in the activities that you usually do together, and you'll feel lonely if he goes ahead without you. Your marriage may become stressful, but this could also be an amazing opportunity to strengthen your bond. Get creative when it comes to romance: you can still have a romantic dinner in bed, watch a movie together, and exchange massages. You might just have to learn the delicate art of feather caressing him, while he can rub all your sore muscles that have had reduced activity. There is usually no restriction on kissing. You can still wear something sexy and have fun coming up with games to keep your love and intimacy going. This is a great time to practice giving unconditionally as well. However, if you really don't feel like having sex, be very frank with your

partner. Some men will be supportive and some will have difficulty with this one. Communication is key here. Speak freely about your frustration and allow him to voice his as well, but don't waste time whining as soon as he comes in the door. That will not bring positive returns. Remember, the power to affect a situation is most often based on how you look at things.

6. Keep fit while in bed. With your practitioner's approval, you could do some exercises in bed such as leg lifts, calf stretches, and upper arm exercises with light weights. Exercising helps promote circulation, as well as keeping your muscles, including your heart, in shape. Make sure you do some breathing exercises as well. Open your window daily and take ten deep breaths, counting to ten as you inhale, then hold for the count of ten, and finally exhaling for the count of ten. Breathing deeply this way will keep your lungs in shape, your blood oxygenated, and your spirit high.

7. Pamper yourself. Staying in bed does not mean denying yourself all the pleasures of life. Hire a massage therapist or ask a friend to give you a head to toe massage at least once a week. See if your hairdresser will come to your bedside. Ask a girlfriend over and have a manicure and pedicure party. Start a book club and invite friends over for an animated conversation. If you have a grandma or an aunt who loves playing a good game of cards, invite her over to play and ask her to tell you some good stories about your mom or dad. Don't give up and spend all day wallowing in the "Why me?" mode. Think of what you would do for your child if she was put on bed rest for months—how you would support her, how you would cheer her up. In fact, that is exactly what you are doing and whom you are doing it for.

8. Bond with your baby. Many women on prolonged bed rest face a dilemma. Though this would seem an ideal time to contemplate the miracle of pregnancy and to really bond with the baby, the usual reason for being on prolonged bed rest is a degree of risk to the baby and the pregnancy. Remember that the vast majority of women who are confined to bed go on to deliver babies who survive and thrive. And for the few who don't, it is doubtful they ever regret loving the little person who was even briefly part of their lives.

9. Get support. Ask your practitioner to give you the phone numbers of other mothers similarly confined to bed rest. Sometimes you can talk each other through a particularly boring day. Contact support groups and visit www.sidelines.org, which maintains a national hotline of volunteers who offer support and match you with other bedridden moms-to-be. This group was started by a California mother who was confined to bed during her high-risk pregnancies. She figured out a way to use her free time for the good of other women in similar circumstances.

10. Get creative. Get colored pencils and paper and draw your feelings. Frida Kahlo learned to paint during a long bed stay and went on to become one of the most celebrated female painters of all time. A lot of her work is self-portraits. Her father had hung a mirror over her bed so that she could copy her own face. You can turn anything that comes your way into a positive experience. If you don't feel comfortable with your ability as a painter, paint anyway, or write. Anthony Robbins says, "A life worth living is worth recording." These art works will be a wonderful way to look back at this period with tenderness.

11. Last but not least, forget about yourself and help others. You can volunteer to do some phone work for a charity. You can be part of a prayer line, help line, or stamp and fold letters for a fundraiser. Call relatives who are sick or alone and cheer them up. Doing service might turn your bed rest into the most fulfilling time in your life.

TAKING ACTION IN THE WORK AND FAMILY ENVIRONMENT

One of the first questions that arises in the first trimester is when you should announce the pregnancy. You may be so excited that you want to tell the world immediately. Or, you may want to wait and cherish the secret. Some people worry about miscarriage and prefer not to tell until its threat has passed. Something to consider, however, is that friends and family can be an enormous source of support in the event of a miscarriage, and you may be missing out on this support by not sharing the news. Talk to your partner about this and do what feels most comfortable for the two of you. Make it a special event whenever you do make the announcement.

You may want to wait to let the people at work know until after the first trimester. Your pregnancy is personal information that you do not need to share until you are ready to discuss your maternity and paternity leave.

FINDING YOUR SUPPORT TEAM

Doulas are sprouting up all over the country and many mothers refer to them as the women who have made their birthing experience special. What is a doula, anyway? A doula is a trained birth coach—a surrogate mother figure who accompanies the couple throughout the entire labor and delivery process. As mentioned earlier, research has shown that with the help of a birth doula there is a much lower risk of Cesarean births, medical interventions, and the use of pain medications.[23] A birth doula's knowledgeable help during delivery produces greater bonding with the newborn. With the help of a postpartum doula, the risk of postpartum depression is also reduced.

Doulas offer what I call a "girlfriend's PIE": Physical, Informational, and Emotional support.

Physical comfort procedures used during labor can include massage, counter-pressure, gentle touch, and literally supporting the laboring woman's body weight during a strong contraction.

Informational support is essential when the labor goes from the comfort of the home to the hospital. Often, as soon as the mother arrives at the hospital, a transformation takes place. She goes from being an empowered birthing mother to a frightened patient. A doula, with her knowledge of the natural physiology of labor and delivery, can explain suggested medical procedures and interventions and help provide the clarity that expectant parents need when faced with medical decisions.

Emotional comfort is crucial if you want to feel safe and secure in the birthing environment. A doula's unique role is to encourage your self-confidence, protect the sacredness of the process, and help you relax and focus on the natural rhythm and progress of your labor.

The next question I usually get is, "How much does a doula cost?" It's hard to put a realistic price on that type of support. I have been at births for as little as four hours, all the way up to twenty-four hours and more. A birth doula also helps the partner experience this magical time with confidence and gives him or her more time to spend with the laboring woman. A doula shows the partner how to help the birthing mother change positions and how to massage her.

She gives the partner a much needed break during a long labor. At home, a postpartum doula helps the partner spend more quality time with his or her significant other and baby by cooking the meals, allowing them to take a nap, and helping the mother with the sometimes challenging task of breastfeeding. She is a loving mentor who shows you ways to appease your baby, bathe, burp, swaddle, and even play with him. A doula is like the village support system revisited.

Today, most women are isolated from the tribe. Many have never seen a birth or seen a woman care for a newborn. Furthermore, some of us have a lot of emotional baggage with our own mothers, and a neutral third party might be just the ticket for your labor, delivery, and postnatal help. Even back in the days when we all lived in the village, it was often a neighbor or a relative who aided women through this life-changing event. A doula brings the village back to where it belongs.

Doulas work hard, and their job is a vocation that comes directly from the heart. Doulas lose sleep so that you can rest, massage your back for hours while you are managing contractions, spoon feed you, wash you, whisper words of encouragement in your ears, help you remember your innate ability to give birth naturally and care for your child, and at times they share your tears or bring you good cheer.

Think of how much you have spent on your honeymoon or the wedding reception. The investment was well worth the importance of the day. The price of a doula is a lot less than those expenses. You've had your honeymoon, now have your babymoon. Now it's time to invest in another important time of your life: your labor, birth, and the first weeks of your baby's life.

If finances are a challenge for you, help is available at a reasonable cost. Birth and postpartum doulas who are going through their certification process charge very little or nothing. They might not have as much experience, but research has shown that just the presence of a compassionate woman is enough to change your birthing experience. Visit www.dona.org to get a list of doulas in your area. For postpartum lactation help, contact your local La Leche League organization. Their counselors often work on a sliding scale, and they offer free peer counselor meetings. Check my Web site www.JoyInBirthing.com for links to international doula associations.

Your baby is worth it, and your investment will prove to have been money well spent.

THE THIRD CHAKRA'S ELEMENT: FIRE

The element of the third chakra is fire. Whereas our first two chakras, earth and water, are subject to gravity and are drawn downward, fire sends its heat and flames upward. We often refer to people as hot-blooded. Others are cold emotionally or physically. Choose the middle way, a balance between the two extremes. This is ideal for well-being, peace of mind, and a harmonious life. Have compassion for yourself this month when your moods seem to swing to and fro like the branches of a tree dancing in the wind.

Light candles at night. If it's winter, cuddle in front of a fireplace, and if it's summer, build a fire at the beach or place a Tikki torch in your backyard and meditate on the flame. This month, surround yourself with laughter, good company, good friends, and funny movies. Go see a comedy show or a musical.

Guided Meditation: Your Birth

As the third chakra represents our self-definition and our identity, it is a good idea to practice the following meditation to heal or embrace your own birthing experience.

Find a place where you will not be disturbed for the next thirty minutes, sit comfortably, and close your eyes. Imagine you are totally relaxed from the tips of your toes all the way up to the crown of your head.

Look for any place in your body that feels tense and let it melt into the chair or sofa you are sitting on. Listen to your breath. With each inhale, allow a comforting glow in, and with each exhale, let go of all your tension. Now imagine a golden white light surrounding you. Take a deep breath in and, as you exhale, see yourself floating in water. It is safe; you are here as a witness and no matter what, you will remember it and you will be able to handle it. Now imagine that you are inside your mother's womb and ask yourself how you feel. Find out what your thoughts and feelings are about your mother and the outside world. If you find yourself in a lot of fear, tell the little one, your unborn self, that today you have come to help her come into this world with love and safety. Tell her that you'd like to accompany her in her birthing journey to discover what happened and to mend or rejoice with her. Tell her that you are here for her and that together you will witness your birth safely and lovingly.

If you can't remember your actual birth, go ahead and imagine the birth you wish you had. Imagine your mother taking you into her arms and welcoming you into this world. It is your right to be here and to have the experience you wish for and deserve. Heal the past or celebrate the actual wonderful birth you had. Once you have gone through the details and have learned much of your own birth, come back up slowly. Use the sound of creation, "Ahhhhh," to bring all of your senses back into your body.

Now open your eyes. It is a good idea to write down what happened. If you remember having a particular traumatic experience, forgive when you can and embrace it with gratitude. Rejoice in the fact that you do not have to inherit your past unless you choose to.

God Has No Grandchildren

One day as I was writing this book, I told a friend that my biggest concern was for my children. "I am simply afraid I will not be able to provide for them," I said, feeling scared and weighed down by the responsibility of single motherhood. "Why are you worried about your children so much?" my friend replied. "Why do you feel it is all on your shoulders? Don't you know that God has no grandchildren? We are all Her children and if She takes care of you, She will take care of them too, directly."

God has no grandchildren. She is the nurturing Mother; He is the providing Father. I don't actually bear all the responsibility for my children on my shoulders alone; I share it with another parent—with Divine Power. Trust your Higher Power to care for you and your child.

MONTH

4

the right to love and be loved

I love, I am loved, and I am lovable. I am in balance. I own my right to be, to have, and to want now. I am open to receiving all of my goods. I know it is God's pleasure to bring to me what is mine by Divine right. As I learn to love unconditionally, I give birth to a loving soul. I am madly in love with the universe and everyone in it. In gratitude and thanksgiving, I release this into the activity of the Law. It is done, and so it is. Amen.

YOUR BABY NOW

Your baby is now about the size of an avocado, about four and a half inches long, crown to rump, and weighing approximately three ounces. In the next three weeks, he'll go through a tremendous growth spurt, doubling his weight and adding inches to his length. The nervous system is starting to function. The reproductive organs and genitalia are now fully developed. At the beginning of your second trimester, you find yourself centered and stronger. You are less tired and most of the early queasiness is gone. This month, you may notice some changes in your skin. Your nipples may darken, and your veins may be more noticeable. Your uterus has outgrown your pelvis and has moved to the abdomen, which will decrease your lung capacity, and you might experience shortness of breath. Your baby's love is taking your breath away.

THE FOURTH CHAKRA

The forth chakra sits on your heart center and represents your right to love and be loved. In the fourth month, the baby is defining its gender; the sexual organs are now formed, and the baby will officially enter into one of the two human tribes: male or female. The love that was experienced for the entire universe at first is being redefined by the baby's sexuality. Even if this definition will be dormant for a few years, the seed for intimate relationships is sprouting. Cell biologist Bruce Lipton, Ph.D., often says in his lectures, "At every level and every stage of development, there is either love and with it, growth—or fear, and with it protection and a thwarting of growth." The fourth chakra is the home of love given and received. It represents the balance point between your physical experience in the first three lower chakras, and the doorway to the connection with the intangible aspects of your character in the five chakras above. Through love, we can transcend the basic animal needs represented by the lower chakras. Love is what connects us to the Divine, and love is what will bring this baby into this world painlessly. By learning first to love ourselves and the Divine, we can intimately love another human being unconditionally. You are learning how to truly follow your heart. To do so, you must first reclaim your right to love and be loved.

EVOLUTION OF THE RIGHT TO LOVE AND BE LOVED

In utero, the baby's needs are fulfilled instantly and automatically. Without asking, the child is constantly soothed by the rhythmic beat of his mother's heart, fed by the umbilical cord, healed by the mother's immune system, and surrounded by a safe environment. This natural and metaphysical connection generates a primordial feeling. *I am completely loved, I am completely lovable, and I am safe.*

But even in the best case, once the baby is born and is growing, parents cannot maintain his original feelings of total safety. Laden by the inevitable circumstances of life, work, money, anxiety, or sickness, parents don't always understand the baby's needs, nor can they anticipate or meet every demand. Every unmet need generates a degree of fear and pain, and the child defaults into immature coping mechanisms. She screams or cries to get attention. She withdraws and becomes aloof or turns into a people pleaser.

Research scientist Bruce Lipton, Ph.D., explains how a child learns behavioral patterns: "A child's brain can download experiences at a super high rate of speed. From the moment a child is born through about the first six years of life, she is in a super-learning state. Children learn and assimilate from how we treat them and how we respond to each other." As the baby learns the meaning of love given and received, he is exposed to ways in which love is commonly used by his parents. Sometimes, to restore harmony, her parents use love as a bargaining chip: "If you really loved mommy, you would not scream at her." Love becomes a reward for good behavior: "What a good job you did . . . Daddy loves you so much." It can be withheld in anger: "I am angry at you, you are a bad girl." Love gets tinted with guilt: "You should love Grandma, look at all the presents she got you." It gets religious undertones: "God loves those who obey Him." It is given on a timetable: "Go on and watch some television, Daddy is busy right now." This way the child learns that love can be used to manipulate others, and that at times, love can hurt and cannot be trusted.

Nonetheless, the quandary is immediately abandoned each time the child is enveloped in her mother's embrace. The sweet feeling of Divine love fills her, and she recalls its primordial origin, how she felt in the womb, and how all her needs were met instantly. But alas, another confusing exchange, and love is once more questioned. We all strive to bring back the primordial love from the womb. We want it now and forever more. As we grow and let go of the familial embrace we enter the world and we discover a new world— the world of our peers.

When we enter school and are surrounded by an unfamiliar group of people, we discover that their approval or love becomes instrumental to our happiness. In an effort to fit in and be accepted by the group, and under peer pressure, we learn to love only those who are considered acceptable, right and hip by others. Concerned only with acceptance and validation, we fall for the cool guy in our school, only to find out (through dating him or being rejected by him) that we are completely incompatible. But there is no time to learn and change our ways. We are still on the quest for someone who will reconnect us to the miraculous and unconditional love we experienced in the womb, and we continue our search outside ourselves. We need direction, but there are no classes on this subject.

Straying from our immediate world, we look further for clues in fairy tales, myths, and the media. Here we are introduced to the impossible and rebellious love of Lancelot and Guinevere, Romeo and Juliet, and Jack and Rose, the lovers from *Titanic*. All these tragedies suggest that true love means losing oneself for the sake of the other. So we dream of the knight in shining armor to come and rescue us from the tower of loneliness. We look for a romantic, sensitive guy with perfect abs and an amazing smile and wit, just like the hero in the latest movie. We are on an impossible journey hoping to find *the one*.

As we mature, we hear mentions that we must love ourselves first, but no one bothers to give us the tools to do so. The fleeting memory of the original state of wholeness we felt in the womb lingers in our unconscious. We yearn for that heavenly love that heals us, makes us feel safe, feeds us without being asked, and lulls us without being told. We continue to look outside ourselves waiting to be fulfilled, loved, and saved. When we finally find whoever we think is *the one,* we experience sheer paradise. We notice every little thing they do, all the minuscule idiosyncrasies of their character, and we love each and every one of them. We stay up at night thinking about them, we talk for hours, opening our hearts like never before. We become sexier, happier, and more blissful than we have ever been.

Sadly, as time passes, we begin to notice things we had not really seen before. It turns out our partners have qualities we can't stand. We expected them to have psychic powers and know what we need or want, and to our surprise, they don't. We demand they satisfy all of our needs, even if *we* don't know what they are. This is not the unconditional love we longed for. Where is the flawless human being that understands us, makes us feel safe, and offers the type of love even *we* are unable to give or receive?

When it comes to love, we have become completely dependent on others, yet based on experiences, we no longer trust anyone to really deliver the love we want. Once again, as we did when we were little, we default into immature coping mechanisms and we learn to operate in a codependent manner. Bargaining ensues: "I will behave this way, if you behave this way," or, "I will show you my love if you show me yours."

We manipulate others by placing blame, finding fault, or attempting to control the situation: "I know you love me, but I wish you would tell me more often, or in a more romantic way." This translates as: "I know you love me, but you are not following my script. Therefore, I can't hear you." We attempt to buy our partner's love by showering them with gifts and favors, disguising our manipulation as generosity and altruism. Some of us enmesh and lose ourselves in the relationship. We compromise our values and integrity, or we minimize, alter, and deny our feelings. There are those of us who need to control and offer advice without being asked and become resentful when others refuse our help. Finally, we find gratification when someone cannot live or function without us. It appears that our self-worth has been validated and everything seems under control, but we are still unhappy. With one foot in the past—what we wish this relationship was—and one in the future—thinking about what it could be—we feel insecure. We can never be satisfied because we fail to appreciate what *is*.

When all efforts fail to produce the desired unconditional and celestial sense of love, we resign ourselves to believing that unconditional love is a myth. We suppress our dream of the idyllic love and learn to cope with the occasional fighting and the feelings of loneliness we experience in our marriages or committed relationships. Then, one fortuitous day, we become pregnant and once again the amazing unconditional love rushes through our veins. That's when we pick up a book called *Painless Childbirth* and are told that we can have this love we have longed for all of our lives. There are no accidents.

You are finally ready to hear the message that has been whispered into your ears over and over again. Yes, you can have it all, you are loved unconditionally and this love is, as the Koran says, *closer than your hands and feet, nearer than your breath.* It lives in your belly, and it is the pure expression of the Divine. Your child right now embodies the image and likeness of God—infinite and unconditional love.

Become fully aware that the Divine is Love in its purest form, and that it is the most potent power in the universe. Your God/child can satisfy your incredible need, your longing for the unconditional love that nurtured you in the womb. The Divine Mother you are embodying can provide the metaphysical, instant fulfillment that comes from all your needs being met.

Empty your mind and heart of all the rules, the expectations, and the conditions you impose on love . . . and love will fill your soul. In Zen Buddhism, there is a concept called beginner's mind. It claims that the mind should be like an empty rice bowl, for only in this state can the bowl be filled.

When you are willing to accept that what you are searching for is beyond any one person, and what you are yearning for is Divine love, you will be liberated. Your relationships will improve. Feeling loved will no longer depend on someone outside yourself, and you will be whole and complete.

Appreciate and revel at all of nature's creations. Fall madly in love with everyone around you, with your life, your pregnancy, your child, and the eternal *now*. It all comes from the same source: infinite love.

LOVE IS THE UNIVERSAL INTERCONNECTIVITY

Your body is filled with love. Think about it. If your body is injured in any way, the entire system extends love for its healing. Without your conscious help and without a word from your will power, your body is responding and fulfilling your baby's needs. Our cells love one another. Our blood loves the veins it runs through, and it brings sustenance to the lungs, brain, and heart. Our feet love our legs, our hands are in love with our arms, and they all communicate with each other and look out for one another. Just like a tree communicates with and sustains the roots, branches, fruits, and seeds, all our body parts are interconnected in a love dance. As trees depend on the earth, water, and air for their sustenance, so too do the earth, sun, and all the stars in our galaxy depend on each other and on other galaxies. Scientists call this interconnectedness. I call it a true love affair. We are born with an innate right to love and be loved, not just by our mothers, fathers, and family members, but by the entire universe. For love is what connects us to all and what we rely on to thrive in this life and this world.

It is love that connects us to every human being on this planet. Whether we are aware of it or not, we have a secret connection established with the other inhabitants of this planet. Take a look around. You probably have many items in your house that come from other countries. You may have a rug from Afghanistan, an item of clothing from Pakistan, India, or Thailand. Your car runs on Iraqi and South American oil, and has Korean and Vietnamese manufactured parts in it. Your cupboard is filled with utensils and plastic items manufactured in China, pottery made in Mexico. Your pantry and refrigerator have foods imported from around the world. The essence, the love, the handiwork of people you don't know, or even those you have been taught to despise, is already part of your life. It sustains you, it moves you, it covers you, and it surrounds you.

Love has found its way into everything you are. All you have to do is become conscious of it and embrace it. When you realize that you are part of this love story, you'll soon see that everyone and everything belongs in it. In truth, all is one. There is no separation. We are all part of one unique and Divine force that encompasses all that there is. Love is the basic principle of all life. Love is the expansive state of the spirit; it transcends boundaries and limitations. It can only be given truly when it is felt for oneself thoroughly.

LOVING ONESELF

A few years ago on the streets of Los Angeles, a large billboard announced: "Become the one you want to marry." How many times have you heard the cliché, you must love yourself before you can truly love anyone else? But how does one love oneself? Here are some simple exercises that can point you in the direction of self-love. As you read them, pay attention to the feelings that come up.

- Tell yourself, "I love you." My kids often make fun of me because I stop by the mirror and make funny faces at myself. In the past, those faces were usually me checking myself out and making a negative remark. Once I became conscious of that habit, I began switching the remarks with a smirk and gibberish. It took a lot for me not to judge myself, but slowly I began looking at my image and saying, "I love you." Today, I wake up in the morning, look at myself in the mirror, and say "Hi baby, how are you! I love you. Have a good day." During the day, if I catch myself looking into the mirror to check out my outfit before I leave, I make sure to add, "You are so cute." The more I say it, the more I feel it and believe it.

- Write yourself a love letter. If you are especially down on yourself, I suggest you write yourself a love letter every day for thirty days. Post it and send it. It is so much fun receiving love letters daily. It can be just a postcard, a short note, or a three-page romantic letter. The act of committing self-love to paper, and then sending and receiving that love, will benefit you profoundly.

- Think of yourself as a child, deserving of hugs and praises. Take a baby picture of yourself and place it somewhere where you can see it often. Look at that baby and transfer all the love you have to her. Imagine she is your daughter and give her all the attention she needs.

- Pamper yourself. No matter your financial situation, you must find ways to pamper yourself. Get a massage, get your nails done, and take a bath surrounded by candle-light and soft music. Take a wonderful walk at sunset in a romantic place. Take yourself out to lunch at your favorite restaurant. All these activities are better done alone. Learn that keeping your own company is as much fun as sharing it with others.

- Accept compliments. If someone compliments your clothes, resist the urge to respond with, "Oh, this little thing?" Learn how to accept compliments, praises, and gratitude with a simple, "Thank you." Keep a list of the compliments you receive for one whole day. You may be surprised by how many times you are the recipient of another's loving consideration.

- Recognize when you are judging yourself, belittling or insulting your actions, and stop. Part of living consciously is being aware of how you talk to yourself. When I was a little girl, I would often remind myself of some embarrassing moment I experienced in the past and I would feel terrible. Those episodes could have happened weeks, months, or even years before, but it seemed that out of the blue they would invade the present and make me feel rotten. For years, I simply could not stop this pattern. Though I would not do it purposefully, these negative thoughts seemed to surface at the most inopportune times, usually when I was down. As a small child I had created a harsh judge that lived inside my head. My childlike logic had resolved that I would be the first to judge myself so that I might correct myself before anyone else could judge me. Today, I have compassion for that child, and when I catch myself in the old behavior, I say, "What you just did was silly. You are so cute! I know you are scared. Don't worry, I am here, you are safe."

- Affirmations that start with "I am . . ." are powerful tools for self-love. Try one of these: "I am loved, loving, and lovable. I am enough. I am a lover of humanity. I have a loving relationship with myself. I feel fulfilled right here and right now." Make up your own and post them everywhere.

- Ask people to tell you what they like about you. I know this one is tough. Once when I was conducting a transformational workshop, I asked people to pay attention to the positive qualities of one another for the next few days. I encouraged them to see each other or talk on the telephone with one another outside the workshop. At the end of the week, we staged a ritual: as though dead, one person at a time would lie in the middle of the room and the entire group would pronounce their eulogy. Later, one of the participants came over to tell me, "At first it was so difficult to hear all these compliments from everyone. I just wanted to crawl into a hole and hide. Then slowly I relaxed and allowed the love to envelop me. People should have their eulogies when they are alive. How sad we never hear those words before we die!"

- Practice compassion and sacred service. When you enter a room, radiate compassion for all you see. Let go of your fear of judgment, of not belonging, of saying the wrong thing, of being misunderstood or being taken advantage of. To live with compassion is to live with passion. Give of yourself with passion. Help others. When you get involved in some type of service, you will feel tremendously rewarded and your life will be augmented. Find a way to give back, whether it is at your church, a shelter, a school, or a charity organization. Find something to do for others and you'll love yourself for it.

Some of these actions will work well for you, while others may not quite fit. If you have paid attention to your reactions, you know which ones you felt were absolutely ridiculous. Try them first! Where there is resistance, there is a lesson to be learned. Then, create your own list by taking a moment to get quiet and asking yourself, "What can I do to help myself feel more compassion and love toward myself?" Let the answer bubble up from inside you. If you can't hear a clear message, try writing out your question, and then let your pen do the talking. You know best what works for you, and you have great wisdom within.

When your baby is born, you will be able to rejoice at each and every little triumph: his first step, first smile, and first word. Examine yourself as if you were your own mother and revel in your ability to get things accomplished so skillfully, so swiftly, and so effortlessly. Loving ourselves includes loving our body as it goes through the natural changes in pregnancy.

LOVE THE WAY YOU LOOK: WEIGHT GAIN IN PREGNANCY

One of the common concerns of pregnant women is the fear of gaining too much weight. Try not to worry, as most of the weight gained during pregnancy is not fat. Women of average weight should expect to gain twenty to thirty pounds during pregnancy. If you are starting the pregnancy very overweight or very underweight, you may be advised to gain less or more. Use your intuition and take a good look at what you put in your mouth, your mind, and your soul. In other words, healthy and organic food, positive food for thought, and self-love will go a long way no matter what the scale says.

GOOD HEALTH [OF THE UNBORN BABY] DEPENDS ESSENTIALLY ON THE IMAGINATION OF THE MOTHER, OR HER INTERIOR LIFE, HER VIEW ABOUT THE MEANING OF LIFE, AND HER HEALTHY EATING HABITS.

ELEANOR MADRUGA LUZES, M.D., *SCIENCE OF THE BEGINNING OF LIFE*

During the first trimester, you will gain approximately 1 to 1¹/₂ pounds a month. During the second trimester, it's ¹/₂ to ³/₄ a pound per week. The final trimester, weight gain is usually ³/₄ pound to 1 pound per week. Remember, all weights are approximate, and your pregnancy may vary. Here is a breakdown of where pregnancy weight generally goes:

Baby	6$\frac{1}{2}$ to 9 pounds
Placenta	1$\frac{1}{2}$ pounds
Amniotic Fluid	2 pounds
Breast Enlargement	1 to 3 pounds
Uterus Enlargement	2 pounds
Fat Stores and Muscle Development	4 to 8 pounds
Increased Blood Volume	3 to 4 pounds
Increased Fluid Volume	2 to 3 pounds
Total	**22 to 32$\frac{1}{2}$ pounds**

While you do need to increase your caloric intake during your pregnancy, it's important to be sure to eat healthy foods and avoid empty calories from cookies, chips, and sodas when you can. Remember, you are providing your baby's nutrition, and proper vitamin and mineral intake is vital for helping your baby grow healthy and strong. If you have questions about your diet or weight gain, be sure to discuss it with your healthcare provider. Each pregnancy, expectant mother, and unborn child is different. Your pregnancy may not progress according to the information found here, which is based on the average pregnancy.

LOVING OUR PARTNER

So far, we have taken a look at the evolution of love, at the Divine solution to obtain unconditional love, and at the tools to practice self-love. Now we can focus on how to love our intimate partner unconditionally.

By now we have hopefully learned that we can't change others—the way they love, the way they act, speak, etc. We know we are the only ones we can transform. We have also learned that our Higher Power is the only source that can fulfill our need and desire for unconditional love. Now, let us look at our present relationships, focusing on what is still unresolved. Look to see if there are any resentments, fears, or negative emotions toward others and yourself.

When we hold resentment for actions taken by others, or when we feel shame and guilt for actions we have taken, we clutter our hearts. Imagine this scenario: three years ago, someone called you stupid, and today you are still holding onto that comment and feeling resentment toward it. You keep recalling the event and each time you do, you get angry at the person who insulted you. Doing so *makes you* stupid for three years. The person who insulted you took three seconds to do the kind of damage you have extended for a very long time. Another example: ten years ago, you hurt a girlfriend by sleeping with her boyfriend, and each time you recall that incident, or even think about her, your insides churn remembering how angry and hurt she was. The action of one afternoon has held you hostage for ten years.

Once we uncover the events done to us and the ones we have perpetrated, we must become ready to let them go. To completely clean house, you must become willing to forgive those who have harmed you and forgive yourself. How would your life be if you forgave the one who called you stupid or forgave yourself for sleeping with your girlfriend's boyfriend—and called her to make amends?

In my experience, after making my own list and calling people from the past to make amends, I discovered that many people didn't even remember what I had done and had held no resentment toward me. Of course, I also found those who took pleasure in adding to my list of wrongdoings. However, instead of becoming defensive, I simply let them vent and when all was said, I felt free and uplifted. I had done my part and had emptied my rice bowl.

Making amends does not mean apologizing. The word was carefully chosen. It means making changes. If I have been insincere with my partner, simply saying I am sorry will not make any difference. Admitting I have been lying to him, promising to myself first and amending/changing my behavior is what is required. If you have been blaming your unhappiness on what others did to you as a little girl, making amends means that you make a commitment to yourself to let go of the resentment of the past, and either heal or let go of the relationships you have with these people. Some relationships, like those with our parents or siblings, are difficult to let go of. Yet continuing to allow those who have hurt you into your life without making any amends/changes is not an option. Unless you let go of all that stands in the way of your serenity, you cannot feel completely loved or completely lovable. Which brings us to forgiveness.

THE ART OF FORGIVENESS

There can be no love without forgiveness. However, this is a very tough action to take. True forgiveness does not mean allowing someone who wronged us to forego his or her rightful punishment. Forgiveness recognizes that the road to happiness lies not in convicting the world of its guilt, but in letting go of our perception of its guilt. In reading the book *A Course in Miracles*,[24] I learned that my anger and blame have made it seem that others were different from me, that I was good and they were evil. Other people's interests appeared to be separate from mine, in competition with mine. In that paradigm, others seemed to be forever seeking happiness at my expense. However, when I looked at my perpetrators with maternal eyes, I saw that their pain and unhappiness were as big, if not bigger, than my own. Forgiveness shows us that other people are the same as we are, with the same needs, the same desires, and the same pain. Forgiveness is a gift we are giving to ourselves, not to anyone else. Forgiveness is something we need to do even before someone wrongs us, even before we meet someone, even before we recognize what we have done to someone else. Forgiveness is at the very foundation of unconditional love.

Forgiveness is not about forgetting, it is about letting go of recreating over and over the same events, the same actions that have been done in the past. Forgiveness is not about erasing the wrong, it is about changing the relationship we have with that which was done to us. It is about letting go of the hold those people and events have on us. Forgiveness is about setting ourselves free.

Cherie's Story

Cherie, a client, once called me to vent. After she had the baby, the father proposed and, shortly after, they got married. Cherie was furious and very hurt by her mother-in-law, Ms. Uppity, because after the wedding, she planned a family reunion and Cherie was not invited. "Why does that woman hate me so much? Why can't she accept I am going to be her son's wife and that we are part of her family?" When I asked her if the grandma had come to see her newborn grandson, she told me that Ms. Uppity only stayed for a very short visit and that the entire time she had tried to take her son and the baby out, with the excuse that "Mom could use a break." I could understand my client's pain and could empathize. She felt righteously indignant. But anger was not going to fix any of it. Cherie asked, "How would love fix this situation?" I suggested she envision her mother-in-law embracing her son at her bosom much like Cherie was doing with her newborn, and to imagine the love that she must have felt for him. I then asked her to realize that something must have gone terribly wrong for a mother not to rejoice in her son's happiness and his new family. We certainly could not speculate on her mother-in-law's circumstances, but we could find compassion, realizing that something must have transpired in Ms. Uppity's life to have manifested such unnatural behavior. I suggested she try empathy and extend her love to her mother-in-law. She would still maintain her boundaries and discuss her feelings with her husband, finding a solution together for the immediate situation. But she would not blame him for his mother's insensitivity and she would find a way to forgive Ms. Uppity, while freeing herself from the emotions that stood in the way of her own happiness.

Remember, forgiving does not mean condoning, it simply means giving up the space resentment has taken up in your spirit. You can be tied down by someone else or by a memory, or you can you can tie yourself down by refusing to let go of beliefs that limit the expression of the whole and complete being that you are. Forgiving can be quite difficult, but nothing goes away by ignoring it. If we wish to grow, forgiveness needs to be implemented. If we can't forgive another, how can we forgive ourselves?

USING LOVE AS A HEALING TOOL

We invite respect or disrespect according to what we give others. All others. Down through the ages, this concept has been referred to in many ways, including *reciprocity*. What we sow is what we reap. We can work in harmony through example and right action to produce an environment that is loving and nurturing for all. *A Course in Miracles* states: "To forgive is merely to remember only the loving thoughts you gave in the past, and those that were given to you."

In Africa, there is a tribe that believes that one way to cure an illness is to concentrate on a part of your body that feels good, and then transfer that feeling to the part that is sick or injured. If you were to twist a wrist, you'd concentrate on the wrist that feels good. You would pay attention to all the little movements, all the sensations of wellness in the healthy wrist, and gently transfer them all to the wrist that was injured. We can apply the same method to our relationships. Make a list of all the things you love about your partner, all the good memories you have of your life together, and embrace the feelings that come up when you recall them. Now all you have to do is transfer this love to whatever area of your relationship you'd like to improve, and then see the law of attraction work for you. Let love mend the disagreements or conflicts you are experiencing. Wake up each morning remembering why you fell in love with this particular person and use that to fuel your state of mind. Use this exercise for every relationship that needs mending.

This exercise will really help you when you are in labor. During the contractions, focus on those parts of your body that feel good. Concentrate on their well-being and harness that sense of relaxation to imbue the next wave that hits your womb. If you stay conscious, you can transfer that well-being into your belly and relax those parts that are working hard to bring your baby into this world.

LOVING MEN

Today, acknowledge the beauty of men. Tell the men in your life you love them. Tell your beloved you know that without him you couldn't have the privilege of experiencing creation firsthand. Tell him how precious his life and his gifts are. Today, acknowledge your husband, your lover, your father, your brother, and every man with whom you come into contact. Celebrate the power of the masculine, whether you are going through this pregnancy alone, with your female partner, or with the man who offered his seed to create this new life. Acknowledge how marvelous the other half of God's expression is.

Let your son know that you will love the masculine in him. Let your daughter know about the magic she can find in men. Tell your child of the respect you have for men, for their power, their strength, their tender caresses, and their vulnerabilities.

A PARTNER'S ROLE

With the advent of the Bradley birthing method, fathers were finally given something important to do. They became coaches for the birthing event. To me, this word diminishes the sacredness of the occasion, and at times is taken so literally that an overtly enthusiastic partner behaves as though he is coaching the World Series. Birthing is not an athletic event, but a deeply loving and sacred experience. The partner's role during labor and delivery is essential to the success of your experience. This being said, my husband was at my side during the birth of my son, massaging and comforting me, while for my daughter's birth, I preferred being completely alone. Understanding the woman's needs and being open to providing what she requires, regardless of what you have prepared for, is crucial.

The nine long months before the actual birth can be a difficult and vague time for the partners in our lives. Partners really have no concept of how we feel physically and emotionally during this time. They need our help and direction to create a safe and friendly environment both for the mother-to-be and the child. They need to feel part of this miraculous process in order to establish a relationship with the unborn child early on. Feelings of fear, worry, and anxiety are common for most new fathers. Our partners are entitled to their feelings. Asking your partner how he or she would like to be involved in the labor and delivery might end up backfiring, as most people's answer to such a question will likely be, "I don't know; what would you like me to do?" This can create frustration for both of you.

One thing I have learned through the years is that if you don't ask for what you want and need, you probably will not get it. Stop thinking he is psychic and assuming, "If he loves me, he'll know what I really need and want." It is unrealistic that your partner will know what you want or need, and such an expectation has nothing to do with love. Giving you what you communicate you want and need, or telling you honestly what he can and cannot give or do, are true expressions of love. So go ahead and ask, trying to be specific. We know by now that one person alone cannot, and never will be able to, give us all that we need. Your partner cannot be the only source of your fulfillment. You must create a support group in this miraculous time. Find friends who are willing to listen and ask your healthcare provider to help you find other mothers-to-be. Find chat rooms and Web sites to answer your questions. Find and hire a doula. Find a therapist if you feel the need to work on some of the tough issues that are coming up. No matter who you rely on, diversify and cultivate multiple sources of support.

Yes, it is your time to get pampered, dear one, but remember that our partners also go through incredible changes during this time. Having a child is an emotional, mental, and spiritual event for both of you. Acknowledge the little and big things your partner does for you. Tell him or her how to be useful. Welcome your partner into your arms as often as you can and remind them why you love them and why you think they will make a great parent. This is such a magical time for both of you, so be sure to cherish it. Every moment counts!

SIMPLE RECIPE FOR A HEALTHY RELATIONSHIP

This has worked for me, but I encourage you to make up your own:

- A daily cup of verbal affirmations of love for your partner and your other children.
- A daily tablespoon of physical loving contact. It could simply be holding hands or a daily hug.
- A daily teaspoon of "I am sorry," with no strings attached.
- A daily ounce of prayer or meditating together, either before dinner or before you go to sleep. If you are not the praying kind, simply recite together a few things you are grateful for. Sharing gratitude can transform your individual life and your life as a couple.
- A weekly date. Make sure it is a weekly affair: a two- to three-hour dinner, an ambling walk, or a bike ride. What you do does not matter. Do it every week, just the two of you. This is a time when you can look into each other's eyes and renew your love.
- Finally, one yearly vacation with your honey, or by yourself, no kids, no responsibilities. If you haven't done it yet, do it before the baby comes.

During your pregnancy, start looking for a trusted babysitter—a reliable grandparent, a neighbor, or a friend who enjoys children. Finding the right person to take care of your baby could take a while, so start right away. Remember, you need time off, your relationship needs time off, and your other children need special time.

You probably think, "When the baby comes, we are not going to want to leave her alone with anyone. I'll be breastfeeding and she'll need me." Yes, at the beginning many parents feel that way, but remember, self-care is important, and cultivating your relationship with your partner is important, too. You will learn how to pump your own milk and have three to four hours off for a date.

If you still think that you can't possibly leave your child in the hands of someone else, start looking anyway. In the event you change your mind, you will have someone there for you.

This recipe is sure to bring you closer to your partner. Now, close your eyes and remember what it was like the first time you felt that love was in the air.

Love Is in the Air

I look for places where I can feel that love is in the air. Sometimes I go to the arrival gate at the airport just to bask and be in the presence of love. Looking at people's eyes in expectation of their loved one returning from a trip, their hearts racing, searching through the crowd for the beloved. Anticipation is boiling like water in a kettle and at the instant of recognition, the whistle sounds and love simply explodes. Some run to each other, for love can no longer wait. It has no age, no sex, and it is not only for lovers. It flows from father to daughter, from cousin to aunt, friend to friend, grandma to child, and husband to wife. Pure, unaffected love. The waterfall of kisses cascading on lips, cheeks, heads, and hands. Sturdy, solid hugs taking the breath away, the joy spilling onto the floor and splashing up to the ceiling, the penetrating looks of these ineffable moments. Love is in the air, and I breathe deeply and let it in.

Another favorite place of mine is the park or the beach, where lovers come together and rekindle their childlike innocence. They play, roll around on the grass or in the sand, laugh, kiss, or simply rest and take in the sun on their lover's bosom. Discreetly I watch them, not wanting to disturb the moment. I simply feel that love is in the air and breathe it in.

Yet, the most magical place I find love is in the delivery room. Yes, the love that rushes headlong out of mom's and dad's hearts at the site of the little one is the most pure, the most Divine love I witness.

At childbirth, parents discover yet another realm of uncharted love in their hearts. A state that is purely Divine, when you know you are willing to give up your life for the loved one without a doubt or a second thought. "Love is in the air," I whisper to the nurses and doctor, and then I breathe in deeply.

THE FOURTH CHAKRA'S ELEMENT: AIR

The element we explore in the fourth chakra is air. This month we learn how to use our breath to regulate our state. As you breathe, your baby breathes with you. Find a quiet place where you will not be disturbed for the next thirty minutes. Sit or lie down and close your eyes.

Guided Meditation: Birthing a Baby

Take a deep breath in, and as you listen to your breath, allow yourself to go deeper and deeper into a state of total relaxation. That's it. Inhale deeply all the way into your belly. See your child feel the breath of fresh air coming from you. With each exhale, let all the stress and all the tension out. Take a few breaths this way and notice that as you breathe, you are becoming more relaxed. Take another deep breath and let all of your thoughts pass through your mind.

Totally and completely relax all the muscles of your body, from the tips of your toes up through the trunk of your body. Take another deep breath and feel the energy spiraling up your spine, relaxing all your tiny muscles up your back and between your shoulder blades and your shoulders. Now pull the energy up to your throat, swallow once hard, then relax all the muscles in your face: around your mouth, your eyes, your ears, in your forehead, and all around your head.

Now feel yourself being surrounded by a golden white light, the white light of creation. Outside of that white light, visualize a green light representing earth, and love, and the spirit of Nature.

Imagine now that you are in a beautiful place. Search inside the depths of your memory for a location where you have been in your past, or a place you have seen in a movie, or read about in a book. A place where you can feel happy, safe, relaxed, and at peace. It could be a beautiful meadow or a sunny beach. It could be on top of a mountain with valleys covered by snow, or it could be at someone's home where you felt most happy, safe, and loved. Search deeply or make it up. Wherever it is, I want you to go there and feel with your entire being the peace and happiness of being there. Now that you are there, look around and notice all the little details of this place. Listen to the sounds that surround you, notice the smells, and sense how the light feels on your skin. Look at the colors, the shapes, and the shadows of this place. Feel all the joy, the happiness, and the power you have in this safe and peaceful place.

Now, remember that inside your very being there is the power of creation. All women for millions of years have been given the knowledge of birthing. We have been given all that we need to bring another human being into this life effortlessly, naturally, and joyfully. Your mother, grandmother, great-grandmother, and all the women who have come before you have gone through this passage before. You have within yourself all their knowledge, their strength, and their abilities. You have all that you need to be successful in your birthing experience.

You are now going to go to your heart center, the core of total relaxation. In order to do this, you will need to imagine that you are walking down a set of stairs. You feel comfortable and secure on them. You know they are leading to your powerful heart center where you will gain the ability to control all the physical sensations that go through your body. You will walk down slowly, and with each step you will get closer and closer to a state of total relaxation. A beautiful golden light is at the bottom of the stairs. It is warm, inviting, and very, very safe. It promises comfort, love, acceptance, and strength.

Imagine now that you are at the top of the stairs. Look around and feel the comfort of the environment and its safety. Now begin the descent. Repeat the following words.

1. I am beautiful and lovable.
2. I am kind and loving, and I have a great deal to share with others.

Feel your body getting lighter and lighter as you take another step.

3. I am talented, intelligent, and creative.
4. I am growing more and more attractive every day.
5. I deserve the very best in life.
6. I have a lot to offer, and everyone recognizes it.

The warm golden light is getting closer, you feel safe and at ease, and you feel welcomed as you take another step.

7. I love the world and the world loves me.
8. I am willing and ready to be happy.
9. I am a good mother and I know all I need to know to bring this child into the world.

Now the light warms your entire body. A beautiful woman is at the bottom of the stairs. She welcomes you with open arms, with love and understanding.

10. I am ready to be a mother to my child.

You are now at the heart of total relaxation. The Mother has welcomed you; she will guide you, protect you, and hold your hand.

Ask the Mother if there is anything that stands in the way of a natural, painless birthing experience. Listen as you pay attention to your breath. Whatever image or memories come up, go with them. Remember, you are now in the witness role, and anything that you see or experience will not impact you emotionally. Trust this process and allow your body and soul to tell you what you need to work on. Dwell in this place as long as you want, and when you are ready, count backwards from five to one and come back into the room. Open your eyes.

You can ask someone to read this meditation to you, or you can record it and listen to it as you do this exercise.[25] Once you come out of this meditation, write down what happened, what you saw, and how you felt. Do this exercise often to clear and reveal to yourself all that is embedded in your unconscious and all that you can learn on the path to a joyful birthing experience.

A Love Letter

One day you showed up in my life. You had been there all along, but I did not see you. I was looking for what was missing instead of finding all that was there. My celestial love radiated out and we were lifted to paradise, the place where I am complete on my own, and together we complete the universe. Our love will be magnified with the birth of this child, at his first smile, at her first step, and again and again. I look deep into your eyes and see the darling child I cradle in my womb. You and I will be together, forever flowing in our child's blood. You and I joined together in eternity in our children's children. You and I joined forever in our Divine legacy. I feel blessed by you, I feel enriched by you. I love you, dear . . . and I feel complete with you.

MONTH

5

the right to speak and to hear the truth

I harness the remarkable power of the spoken word and use it with purposeful intention. I speak my truth respectfully, and I am willing to be teachable. I listen to the words I hear and learn from them. I commit to speak only when my words are true, necessary, and loving. In gratitude, knowing that successful communication is achieved, I give life to a world leader. I release this word onto the creative sound waves of the universe, and I let them be. It is done. Amen.

YOUR BABY NOW

Your baby now weighs about three-quarters of a pound and is approximately ten and a half inches long. The eyebrows and eyelids are fully developed, and fingernails cover the fingertips. A protective coating called vernix caseosa[26] begins to form on the baby's skin. By the end of this month, your baby will be about eleven inches long and will weigh almost a pound. You might have already experienced your baby move, or you may just be starting to feel it for the first time. Babies tend to be more active when the mother slows down and relaxes. When the mother is active, the movement of the pelvis rocks the baby to sleep. Your partner will get excited when he feels the baby move under his touch. If you have not started yet, talk to your baby every day and encourage your partner to do the same.

THE FIFTH CHAKRA

The fifth chakra, located in the throat, is the center of communication and creativity. Here we learn our right to speak and hear the truth. There is a definite correlation between the movement of the baby and the beginning of communication between parents and child. Finally the baby is no longer only a lump in the mother's belly or a heartbeat we hear at the doctor's or midwife's office. The baby is communicating with the world outside by kicking the mother's belly and saying hello. Our partners or other children get really excited and begin communicating with the baby as well. The fifth chakra potential is fully exploited when we learn how to communicate using our heart and conscious mind together. By allowing only our hearts to speak, we forfeit the use of our consciousness and at times fail to take advantage of our acquired knowledge. In other words, we unconsciously react from our emotions and fail to take into consideration what *is*.

When we only use our mind, we are more interested in being right and at times forfeit the truth to protect our righteousness. Conscious living is embracing and expressing the truth of what is in a loving way. The truth resides in the eternal here and now. There is no such thing as *your* truth, but only *one* truth, and that is the Universal truth. The Greek philosopher Plato said, "Truth is the beginning of every good thing, both in heaven and on earth; and he who would be blessed and happy should be from the first a partaker of truth, for then he can be trusted." When we balance our conscious mind with our heart and are willing to stand for the truth, we are ready to own our right to speak and hear the truth.

THE RIGHT TO SPEAK AND HEAR THE TRUTH

As stated in Article 19 of the Universal Declaration of Human Rights, "Everyone has the right to freedom of opinion and expression; this right includes freedom to hold opinions without interference and to seek, receive, and impart information and ideas through any media and regardless of frontiers."[27]

It is our natural born right to speak and hear the truth. Following the barbaric acts witnessed by the world in World War II, an assembly of several countries got together to create an international document to uphold this right. Still, this freedom is limited in many countries, cultures, and even in many families.

> THEY WHO KNOW THE TRUTH ARE NOT EQUAL TO THOSE WHO LOVE IT, AND THEY WHO LOVE IT ARE NOT EQUAL TO THOSE WHO DELIGHT IN IT. ONE WHO DELIGHTS IN TRUTH MANIFESTS THE QUALITIES OF BEING TRUE: GENUINENESS, FAITHFULNESS, HONESTY, EXACTNESS, CORRECTNESS, AND RIGHTEOUSNESS. HE IS LEGITIMATE; FIRM OR STEADY IN ADHERING TO PROMISES. HE IS WORTHY OF TRUST.
>
> CONFUCIUS

Freedom of speech scares those who wish to maintain the status quo, who are afraid to go against the grain, or simply can't deal with someone else's opinion. Interestingly enough, children are born embodying this right.

Children are born incapable of lying. As soon as they are able to express themselves, they rejoice in sharing the truth about their likes and dislikes, and naturally expect the world to be true. If you want an honest opinion, ask a toddler. They never lie until they are taught differently. As they grow, kids are trained to curtail their words, even with those they trust. For example, a child tells his mother, "Mom, I don't like Uncle Charlie, I don't want to go to the park with him." Mom replies, "What are you talking about? He's your uncle. Be nice and don't you let me hear you say that again." If you observe a child's first reaction to this kind of response, you will notice a startled expression. His eyes open wide, and his appearance is one of surprise. His mind is trying to compute the unnatural concept that the truth is not always acceptable. He struggles with a quandary: When mom asks if I like the juice she gives me, she wants me to tell her the truth, but when it comes to Uncle Charlie, she wants me to tell a lie. When should I tell the truth? After a few more exchanges of this kind, the child learns to put on a false front. A new question lingers: if I have to lie about what I like or dislike, what are the guarantees that others aren't lying to me? What's left is a confusing message: sometimes, you cannot speak the truth, you cannot trust others to speak their truths, and even your parents don't want to hear the truth. With such a mixing of messages, the trust we were born with is jeopardized.

Understanding our environment is vital to our growth. Knowing whom to trust and when to trust can determine whether you'll live a life in fear or confidence.

TRUST BEGINS IN THE WOMB

The connection the mother and child share during pregnancy is so intimate and close that the emotions and thoughts experienced by the mother are directly felt by the child through hormonal and chemical shifts in the body. Bruce Lipton, Ph.D., in an article entitled *The Wisdom of Your Cells* points out, "Blood contains all of the information molecules, such as hormones and emotional chemicals. The mother is always adjusting her physiology and her emotions to deal with the contingencies of life. Since her blood via the placenta is directed to the fetus, the fetus is experiencing and feeling what the mother senses. When stress hormones cross the placenta, they have exactly the same target sites in the fetus as they have in the mother."[28]

Psychologist Erik Erikson's stages of psychosocial development suggest that trust and mistrust are the first building blocks of personality. According to Erikson, choosing one versus the other, trust or mistrust, is the result of our first learned experiences in the womb.

The development of trust and mistrust continues into the toddler and childhood years. The level of reliance your child will feel in her life is correlated with your ability to keep your word and allow her to freely express herself with you. As a mother, you represent the safe haven the child can rely on and return to when going out and exploring the world. You are the one person she was born to trust unconditionally and the one whose job it is to teach her the art of speaking and hearing the truth.

Regardless of what we have been taught as children, today we have a greater responsibility as adults and parents to learn to be conscious of our words. When we pass our own words through the sieve of, "Is it true, necessary, and loving?" we teach our children how to use words consciously.

For instance, to tell Uncle Charlie, "I don't like you," is true, but it is neither necessary nor loving. To tell Uncle Charlie, "I'd rather not go to the park and play right now," is a loving way to enforce a boundary. Often clients that enter the hospital during labor want to make sure the nurse will follow their Birth Plan, and they will either try to explain to her why they chose not to have an epidural, which often leads to a sparring of opinions, or they get irritated and get into a screaming match with the nurse who does not want to cooperate. Sometimes nurses, in an effort to help you, will insistently offer what they believe is the best remedy to a laboring woman: drugs. They mean well, and once you are hooked up to all the gadgets they have to offer, they can perform their jobs better. They can monitor you from another room or from the nurses' station and don't have to work so hard to keep checking on you. Of course, it is your right not to have pain medication offered constantly, and it is the right of a woman to ask not to be given unsolicited advice such as, "You don't have to be a hero, sweetheart. Every woman does fine with an epidural. Trust me." Yet, we still need to learn how to pass our words through the filter of, "Is it true, necessary, and loving?" Certainly it is true you don't want an epidural, but it is not necessary to tell the nurse why, nor is it necessary for her to understand your reasoning. Now all you have to do is focus on loving. When asked, a simple "No, thank you, please don't ask again," will do.

KEEPING YOUR WORD

Telling the truth and keeping your word belong in two different categories. Some people are really careful with their words. Others speak without thinking. I remember when I would promise my children a reward for an accomplished chore, they made sure I kept my word. Children put a lot of weight on our words and they depend on our promises. Keeping your word is essential to building trust in yourself, your relationships, and your life. It is not only good for you, it also sets a good example for the child in your life. You can't change how other people use their words, but you can become conscious of your own.

IF WORDS WERE CURRENCY, HOW RICH WOULD YOU BE?

I invite you to shift paradigms for a minute and look at your everyday words as bank notes. If you treat your words as your currency, your hard cash, would your vocabulary change? You wouldn't squander your money thoughtlessly. You wouldn't waste your money on people who don't deserve it. You would not bankroll an enemy by spending a lot of words talking about them. What about other people's words? When you view their words as money given to you to carefully safeguard, you wouldn't spend it behind their backs by sharing it with strangers or through gossip. When you make a commitment to someone,

> BE IMPECCABLE WITH YOUR WORD. SPEAK WITH INTEGRITY. SAY ONLY WHAT YOU MEAN. AVOID USING THE WORD TO SPEAK AGAINST YOURSELF OR TO GOSSIP ABOUT OTHERS. USE THE POWER OF YOUR WORD IN THE DIRECTION OF TRUTH AND LOVE.
>
> DON MIGUEL RUIZ,
> *THE FOUR AGREEMENTS*

and you have given them your word, imagine that you have given them a bank note to redeem at a specific time.

A kept promise to your loved ones can be as valuable as a million bucks. The more challenging the promise, the higher the reward. Make sure your currency is worthy. Harsh words, sarcastic words, and hurtful words are counterfeit currency. The big bucks are in encouraging words, compassionate words, and loving words. The more you invest, the more you'll receive. Promise yourself to change something you are not happy with, and do it. Now that's priceless.

THE TRUTH ABOUT BEHAVIOR MANIPULATION

When we long for love, attention, or appreciation, we implement a learned strategy to achieve our goals. We use words and behaviors to manipulate others and satisfy their needs.

WHO YOU ARE SPEAKS SO LOUDLY, I CAN'T HEAR WHAT YOU SAY.

RALPH WALDO EMERSON

Some people are always angry. They complain about everyone and everything. They have learned that their best defense is to attack, and they are constantly looking for drama, searching for what is wrong. This state makes them feel safe, for if everyone is focused on the world and how bad things are, no one will focus on them.

It is similar for those people who are always sad; they take on a passive-aggressive stance so that the people around them will work hard at trying to convince them that things are not as bad as they feel. In essence, they need others to tell them everything will be OK. Fear runs their lives, and the only consolation is to constantly have someone reassuring and comforting them. Our society is very good at that. All you need to do is notice how many people rally at your side when you are down and depressed, and how many have no time to rejoice with you for an accomplishment. As a society, we tend to reward pain and suffering more than strokes of luck, genuine accomplishments, and good fortune.

At the opposite end of the spectrum, there are the jokesters, those who are fun to be with, always have something comical to say, and constantly make fun of everything. For those folks, it's our laughter that cuddles them and tells them they are accepted.

All these strategies are based on the need we have for other people's approval in order to feel good about ourselves. We have yet to learn how to talk to ourselves and listen to our Higher Power to regain the primordial trust we felt prenatally. Living in a world we have learned to distrust, we use the behavior manipulation we learned in the very early stages of our life.

Here are two stories that illustrate how once we change our patterns of communication and our automatic reactive behaviors, we can live a fuller life.

Clients' Stories

Sharon: "When I cried, my parents fought. One wanted to console me, the other wanted me to learn how to deal with my emotions on my own. Mom was a firm believer in the philosophy that children need to learn how to self-soothe, self-entertain, and self-pacify. Even though I loved my father, and loved when he rescued me, I longed for my mother's affection. I made this unconscious pact: I will try to never cry, and when I do, I'll hide it and suppress it. This has led to today's consequences: when people cry, I am in fear and get irritated, and usually leave the room in a huff. People tell me I am an angry person, and that I have no compassion. The truth is that I am afraid that, if I stay and witness someone else's distress, all the feelings I have suppressed for so many years will come tumbling out. I have this image of getting lost in my tears forever. I want to have an epidural because I am afraid of the emotions that will surface during labor. This awareness has led me to take the following actions to achieve my desired natural childbirth. Actions I can take today: I have decided to hire a doula to be there in case I lose control of myself during labor. I will do the work I need to do to let go of the past. I will write a letter to my mom and dad and tell them how I felt when I was a baby. I will not send the letters; they are for me and my own healing. I will visit my child-self before I go to sleep and tell her about her right to feel her feelings. I will welcome tears if they come up and will allow myself ample time to let them flow. I've printed my affirmation on little address labels and have affixed them all over the house. If I feel scared or fearful, I will repeat my affirmation silently in my mind until I feel safe. My daily affirmation is: "I am a loving and compassionate person. I am capable of managing my emotions, and it is safe to share them with my partner and my doula. I am safe."

Jenny: "When I was born, I was taken away and placed in an incubator. Mom stayed home, and when Dad came to visit, he tapped on the glass but was not allowed to touch me. Pact: I am not wanted, I am alone, I am not good enough to be touched and loved. Today's consequences: I have a hard time with intimacy. When I make love to a man, I fall apart. I get so attached to him, I suffocate him. I am in constant fear I will lose him. I want a child, but can't seem to find the right person. I am often depressed and sad. Actions I can take today: I will go slowly when entering a relationship. I will wait before I get involved intimately, until I feel safe. Before I take any actions, I will check my underlying emotions. If I feel strongly one way or another, I will wait for an hour, a day, a week, or a month before I take that particular action. My affirmation: "I am a loving person. People want to know me and be with me. I am safe."

THE THREE S'S

In order to break recurring behavioral patterns, we have to take a conscious look at them as they appear. At first you might not be aware of them, but slowly, the more you commit to living consciously, the more you'll begin noticing your patterns. That's when you are ready to implement what I call the three S's: **S**top, **S**hake it off, and **S**tart all over again.

When you catch yourself reacting negatively to a person or situation:

1. *Stop* what you are doing or saying. Leave the room and go for a walk, even just a few steps away will calm you and change your state.

2. *Shake it off.* Forgive yourself, without harsh self-judgment, for the behavior or words you've spoken. If the words came from someone else, still follow step one. Simply state, "This conversation is triggering me. I need a minute." There is no need to accuse anyone. Shake off the feelings that have come up. If the feelings are really strong, as you walk around or take a shower or bath, do the Emotional Inventory Exercise to see why your reaction is disproportionate to the occasion.

3. *Start Over.* After you are sure you have changed your state, become willing to start over. We usually do this either by making amends for what we have said, or by sharing what we've just experienced. It is a good idea to go through the list of why you love whoever triggered the emotion as you cool off or you'll find yourself recounting all the wrong things they have done in the past, which will only add fuel to the fire.

It might be really helpful to recite the serenity prayer: "God grant me the serenity to accept the things I cannot change, the courage to change the things I can, and the wisdom to know the difference."[29]

THE SOUND OF CREATION

The element represented in the fifth chakra is sound. In the Eastern philosophies, mantras or chants are often used during meditation to reach a state of transcendence. When we meditate, our minds can go into chatter and it can be very difficult to stop it or silence it. I've found that chanting a mantra during meditation helps me focus.

During the birth of my daughter, I discovered the sound *Ah*. This sound is used as a mantra in one of the most ancient forms of meditation. In India, it is believed that *Ah* is the first sound of creation, the root mantra and primal sound with which all creation issues forth. Dr. Wayne Dyer, who made this chant popular in the early nineties, noticed a common denominator between this sound and the sound we make when pronouncing the many names given to the creator. See for yourself by saying these out loud: God, Atman, Ra, Buddha, Tao, Krishna, Allah, and Yahweh. All these names have one sound in common, the sound *Ah*. People refer to the "ah-ha" experience when they talk about a moment of sudden insight or discovery, the sudden finding of a solution to a problem. *Ah* is what we say in the moment of ecstatic conception. *Ah* is what we exclaim when we feel satisfied, when we finally exhale. *Ah* is the sound of creation.

In labor, the sound *Ah* is instrumental for two purposes: it will guarantee you'll keep a rhythmic breath, and it will give voice to the feelings you are experiencing. The sound should come from a very low point in your body. In fact, it should generate right at your uterus and move up through all the chakras until it reaches above your head and transports you into the sacred place of creation. If done properly, your body will not be able to tense up while chanting. Chanting the sound *Ah* keeps us aligned with the universe, our body, and our child.

Here is how you can practice it. Find a time in your day when you can comfortably sit undisturbed for at least twenty minutes. Close your eyes and take a deep breath in. As you exhale, float with the sound of *Ahhhhhh*. When you make the sound, place one hand on your belly and feel the sound as it resonates into your uterus. Make sure the sound does not come from your throat, or it may get sore.

Now continue to chant *Ahhhh,* and imagine the wave of a contraction arising in your body. Ride it with the sound, as you would ride a wave, and relax in between, envisioning your cervix opening up like a flower. You will notice that as you vocalize the sound *Ah,* you cannot tense up your body—it brings total relaxation.

Usually, when we are fearful we hold our breath. As we do this, all our muscles tense up and pain increases. With the profound sound *Ah,* you will create a clear channel from your ninth chakra, down through your entire body, and out of your first chakra, encouraging your baby to come forth.

Sit comfortably, close your eyes, take a deep breath and begin your *Ah* meditation. Do it every day until you give birth. Become an expert at relaxing every single muscle of your body.

The Power of the Spoken Word: Susan' s Story

Susan wanted a natural birthing experience. She had witnessed her sister's drug-free, natural birth and wanted the same for herself, but she did not think she could pull it off. She kept saying that she'd try, but she might have to ask for pain medication because she was not confident in her own ability to manage. She was constantly questioning her decisions and felt very ambivalent about her instinctual desire to have a natural and drug-free birth. She needed to change her internal dialogue. Here is how she found the words she needed to obtain her desired birth:

"What originally happened at a very young age, three to five or so, is that I started going to Christian Science

Sunday school. I didn't believe in what we were being taught, even then. I felt alone, trapped, and kept going along with it on the outside, but felt distant the whole time I was involved in religion until I was fifteen years old. This was my first experience with being unable to make a decision. My mother was a CS follower and my father was not. We were always asked to choose, when sick, whether we wanted to pray to heal ourselves or go to the doctor. It was like choosing between Mom and Dad . . . I would always hedge my bets and not really decide. I'd pray with Mom, then if I got super sick, my Dad would insist I be hauled off to the doctor.

"I felt distant, trapped, unsure, ambivalent, not invested, critical. This is what I came to believe: that limbo was better than making a decision. This is what is happening today as a result of my belief: I will do all the research and work hard and then abandon it before making a real decision. I feel unworthy of making life-changing decisions. The affirmation that can help me is, 'Thank you, God, for helping me feel worthy and capable of making important decisions.'"

In the last few weeks leading to her due date, Susan went to a couple of acupuncture treatments where she spoke to her baby and encouraged her to come when the time was right. Her husband called me one evening around 8:30 p.m. Susan was having contractions that lasted about forty-five seconds every ten minutes. They just wanted me to know, as they were getting ready to take a walk around the block. They had run around all day getting last minute things done. It sounded like they had been nesting[30] all day and that Susan had distracted herself from her early labor contractions until her and her husband had finally come home and sat down for dinner. Here's the rest of the story written by Susan:

Susan's Birth

My doula, Giuditta, arrived at just the right moment. We needed her. The contractions were getting really strong and we were having a little bit of a hard time finding a position that would work for me. My doula got me to slow my breathing down during my contractions so that I could manage them better. We tried my sister's hold for a few contractions. [Susan had helped her sister a year ago have a natural, drug-free birth, and was very much attached to using the same position her sister had used. She wanted me and her husband to hold her by the rib cage, so that she could surrender all her weight onto us and go limp.]

After a few times, my doula suggested that I try to lie down on the bed and relax. I was really worried about doing that. The contractions were intense enough that I just didn't believe I would be able to survive that way, but my doula said I should give it a try. I needed to rest. I wasn't sure. I felt scared. I was worried that the pain would be more intense if I was lying flat on my side, not able to move. But she said that I was going to exhaust myself by standing through the contractions. She encouraged me to try resting on the bed, and even napping a bit. I didn't believe that it was even possible for me to be able to nap between contractions, but she was right. I lay down and relaxed every muscle in my body that I could. This slowed down how quickly the contractions were coming. I actually dozed off quite a few times between each contraction. Ken was behind me on the bed, touching my back, falling asleep with me and then waking up to breathe with me when a contraction gathered. This felt great. Giuditta sat in a chair in front of me and talked to me, calming me and getting me to focus when a contraction would come. The contractions were really strong. Really strong. I have never felt something like this before. I lay there, limp and loose, and told myself that I could do this. That I could be limp and loose. That I was opening inside, opening for our baby to come.

As the contractions became really strong, my doula would grab my hand and tell me to focus on it, and she'd breathe with me and Ken.

At some point, I felt my entire body shaking. Giuditta asked me if I felt the baby moving. Indeed, I could feel the baby's movement. I felt relieved because then I knew she was OK. I could actually feel her moving down, dropping further into my pelvis.

When I began feeling some rectal discomfort, I knew it was time to go to the hospital. I got concerned about how I would manage the change. Right after a contraction, I got up and walked downstairs to the backseat of Ken's car. Luckily, once again, I made it to lying down without having a contraction. The surges were super strong and intense at this point. I couldn't believe that they could get more intense, but they did! The ride to the hospital was hard, but not impossible. We must have started driving around 11:30 p.m. because I know we arrived around midnight.

On the way, I prayed, "Let go, let go, let go." Giuditta whispered, "Let God, let God, let God." I walked into the emergency room entrance. I was really beside myself. I wasn't really there. I hung onto my doula while she talked to people. I didn't look at anyone or anything. It wasn't that I was upset or anything, I literally just had the focus on one thing: what was happening inside of me. The tremendous earthquakes shaking my core. Moving my center. It took all my focus. I heard everything that was going on around me, but my sight went. I didn't really take in the hospital. I had been worried about the clinical atmosphere of the hospital. I shouldn't have been. I was consumed by my internal world. Nothing exterior made a dent on my inner events.

There was all this commotion about my getting into a wheelchair. I had been warned about this. There was no way I was going to sit down. I guess I was being really loud about my contractions and moaning a lot.

The way we managed the contractions all the way through was to be very vocal. Sometimes, Ken and I would say *yes, yes, yes*, sometimes *ahhhhh, ahhhhh, aahhhhh*. My doula would always try to get me to extend the sound, make it a real release and use it to calm down.

When contractions would come, they consumed my very being and the world outside stopped, except for my hearing. I could hear most everything. I responded to people talking to me. Though I couldn't focus and see in a regular way, I could hear them.

We made it upstairs and into the triage, and I begged to be allowed to lie down. I quickly pulled off my underwear and pants and just dropped them on the floor and climbed on the bed. The contractions were even more intense since we'd had all that activity. Giuditta reminded me of that. She added that they should settle down again as I rested. I lay on my left side. They put monitors on me and I was happy and relieved to hear the baby's strong, healthy heartbeat. We kept moaning through my contractions.

The nurse wanted to check how dilated I was. I was scared that after all we had gone through, I would only be at five centimeters and then I knew I'd be a goner. I'd have to get medication. I just couldn't hack another five hours like this. The nurse said I was eight centimeters! Amazing. They told me I was going to be given a delivery room.

Those last contractions were the most intense of all. Giuditta and Ken kept telling me I could do it. I wasn't so sure anymore. I've never felt anything like that. All I know is labor is the most intense experience I have ever had, the most intense physically and emotionally. I wish I could describe what it felt like. I certainly had to cry out. I couldn't be quiet. I could stay pretty much limp and loose, minus the shaking, which actually relieved the intensity of the contractions somehow. *Aaaaaaahhhhhhh*. I did it. I did it every time. I was out of my head, out of my body. The nurse checked me again and said I was nearly fully dilated, I just had a little lip on one side around the baby's head. I pushed a bit and she checked again and I was fully dilated. As the doctor had not yet arrived, my doula asked the nurse if the midwife was there. She was. She came in a moment. They prepared me to push, telling me what I'd need to do. I had never worked so hard in my life. It felt like I was trying to move a mountain. The spaces between were such sweet relief.

Giuditta kept telling me to enjoy the peace between each contraction. That really helped me sink into them. Enjoy them. Relish them. That helped me focus on the downtime rather than what was coming next. We would wait quietly. I would go limp and loose. I would feel very relaxed. I was told at one point they even heard me snore in between pushes. I would feel a contraction building. We would start. Each time I felt disappointed that she hadn't come out yet, everyone would encourage me to stay in the moment.

Twice, my doula took my hand down to feel the baby's head. The first time, I could feel her head a few inches back in my vagina. The second time was when she was crowning. It felt so strange, all that pressure down there. The ring of fire, I guess it's called. It felt like the ring of intense pressure. So full, so tight, so taut, so needing to come out of me. I think I got her out in less than twenty minutes. It was such a relief to get her out. She was put right on my chest. I heard them talking about Ken cutting the cord. I was blitzed out of my mind and so relieved. I'm very proud of myself now. It was such an intense experience. Slowly, it has sunk in that we are now three. That my belly is empty of baby. That what I did was a fabulous, wonderful thing to be proud of. We got the lucky sevens. Birth date: 7/7/07. In Delivery Room 7. And she was 7 pounds, 7 ounces!

The one thing that helped me most throughout the entire labor and delivery was my affirmation: "Thank you, God, for helping me feel worthy and capable of making important decisions." I kept repeating it to myself over and over again, I guess until I truly believed it."

THE TRUTH ABOUT PAIN

Whenever I start a lecture, I ask the audience of expectant mothers what their most pressing question is. Inevitably, I always hear, "I want to know how I can manage the pain of labor!" And I always tell them, "If you focus on the pain, I guarantee that you will experience it." Focus on the beauty of the moment, the sacredness, and a joyful loving birthing experience will be yours. Create a realm where worry, fear, and pain may not enter.

Birthing is the Divine miracle. See yourself as the vessel through which God is becoming incarnate. Realize that you no longer need to focus on managing the pain of labor. You no longer wish to numb the experience. You will not be fighting pain, for where you are going there is no pain. Where God dwells, there is no pain, no struggle, no worry, and no fear. When God comes to us, within us, and for us, there is only love, joy, and happiness. Yes, it will be intense. Yes, you will feel the pressure of the manifestation.

Be still, do not resist this truth. Let the doctors and nurses exclaim, "Did you see what just happened in that room? That woman, so focused and at peace? She did not seem to be in pain. How can this be? This must be a miracle!" Make it your agency and ministry. This is your mission, your special contribution to this universe, to have a painless and beautiful birthing experience. Don't do it just for yourself. Do it for all women around the world who will learn from and thrive from your example.

WHAT WE LISTEN TO IS IMPORTANT

It is amazing how important what we hear and listen to are to our well-being. When it comes to choosing something to listen to, to prepare ourselves for the birth, I am partial to hypnotherapy, guided meditation, and affirmation tapes. I like the relaxation that comes with closing my eyes and listening to them. I like the positive statements found in them and the relaxation techniques they teach. I have several tapes and usually go to sleep with my headphones on, listening either to how to improve my life, or how to relax each and every part of my body. And yes, I also listen to my own hypnotherapy CDs. I figure it has to work for me if I want it to work for you. I also love music—all kinds of music. Since I have decided to stop watching television, I make use of my stereo by either listening to music, books on tape, or some interesting radio shows.

We also must take a look at what *not* to listen to, or not to pay attention to. Stay away from worrying friends. You know, the ones that are always stressed about something and that like to tell you about all the bad things that are happening, rehashing all the negative stories they hear all the time. It is not only music or the media that can attack your sense of well-being. It is, most importantly, friends and family members. If you are thinking, "How can I not talk to Aunt Martha while I am pregnant, even though when I do, I feel depressed and worried?" Well, it is time to create new boundaries with the Aunt Marthas of the world. If you cannot avoid seeing that kind of friend or relative, tell them that you no longer want to hear the "woe is me" stories, and tell them that you are doing it for the baby. Exercise your right to speak the truth when it is necessary, and you are doing so in a loving way.

Dr. David B. Chamberlain, in his article "Early Parenting," tells us, "Prenates memorize the voices of their mothers and fathers in utero while learning the basic features of their native language, the 'mother' tongue, as we say. Spectrographic analysis of voice and cry sounds as early as 26 weeks of gestation show how far babies of this age have already progressed in adopting the voice characteristics of the mother. In a recent experiment, mothers repeated a children's rhyme daily for four weeks from week 33 to 37 in utero. Tested at 37 weeks while still inside, the babies reacted with a change of heartbeat to the familiar rhyme, but not to an unfamiliar rhyme. The womb turns out to be a stimulating place and is, in many ways, a school."[31] Once again, we are told by studies what mothers have instinctually known for centuries: singing lullabies to their babies during pregnancy will create a primordial memory in the child that will continue throughout his life. When I was pregnant with both my children, I created songs and incorporated their names in them. When I held them in my arms and sang their songs to them, Natascia and Azzurro responded immediately by calming down, smiling, and going to sleep.

SILENCE

When we talk about our right to speak, we cannot forget our right to be silent. In remembrance for someone who has passed on, we are often required to take a few minutes of silence to celebrate their lives. Silence is something that is used out of respect. It is a powerful weapon against verbal abuse, and it is often where God resides. At times, we may have used silence to hurt someone by giving them "the silent treatment." However, that was not true silence, but rather a lack of interaction. In fact, our mind was probably only pretending to be still and silent. When true silence is observed, we can reach a higher state of consciousness.

In the first book of the Torah, it states: *In the beginning, the earth was a formless void.* Out of this void, this stillness, this silence, everything that is, is contained. Silence is within you. It is not just the absence of sound or lack of noise. It is the ground, the basis of your very being. There is nothing to find out and nothing to prove. Just listen with your whole being to what is here, now. In music and the performing arts silence is as important as sound and words. A filmmaker can create an extremely dramatic moment using simply silence. Silence is an amazing and powerful state. It is with you now. It is you. The only way to find this is to stop everything else. Just be! Sometimes in the delivery room of a hospital, as the child is about to be born, there is a lot of commotion. The nurse is giving instructions to the woman on how to push the baby, or is counting to ten to indicate how long one push should last. Then there is the doula reassuring her client, the husband encouraging her, and the doctor or midwife doing his or her part. I have also seen doctors and nurses having a mundane conversation in between contractions to pass the time. The environment is transformed into a loud and often chaotic stage. In order to better concentrate, relax, and have a sense of serenity, it is best to pare the team down. One person should coach you, while your husband encourages and loves both you and baby. Silence is a beautiful and peaceful environment in which to be born, and once the baby is in your arms, silence is highly recommended, for there is no need for words when love is in the air.

Words Are Highly Overrated

When I first got in touch with Olivia, we communicated via e-mail. The job sounded wonderful at first. Olivia was hearing impaired, could only read lips, and could hardly talk. For cultural and religious reasons, she could not use sign language, so we were to communicate only via e-mail. The challenge was that she belonged to a very strict religious sect with many sets of rules that needed to be respected and followed. Some of those rules included that I could never touch or look at her husband straight in the eyes. He could not touch her or look at her naked, so I had to make sure her body was covered at all times while he was in the room. They could not drive on a specific day of the week, and couldn't do many other things on that special day. They were specifically looking for someone not in their religious group to be available to do those things they were not allowed to do.

Olivia could not meet me before the birth. I was not allowed in their home and she only wanted me to be with her at the hospital. I had many mixed feelings about this challenge. The feminist, the equal opportunity advocate, and the freedom of religion representatives that live in my mind were all having a big discussion. That's when my heart went over my head and I accepted the job. I figured we certainly had the most important ingredient in common: the Divine.

Her husband first called me on a Friday at 3:45 p.m. and told me Olivia was contracting every five minutes and lamenting that it was painful. I usually get the woman on the phone to assess her state, but in this case I had to go by my intuition. They rushed to the hospital before sundown and when I met them, Olivia was smiling. When the midwife checked her, she was only four centimeters dilated, 80 percent effaced, and the baby was at a high station. Even though her waters were still intact, they had asked her to stay at the hospital because she was a little overdue. Her husband left us and went to pray. She and I took to the stairs to see if we could help walk this baby down. I welcomed this opportunity to get to know Olivia. She explained that I had to keep on her right for her so she could read my lips. She was a beautiful woman, twenty-three years old, and this was her third baby. She had a lot of energy and exuded self-confidence, she seemed like an old soul in a young woman's body.

By 7:00 p.m., a nurse checked her and said that she was six to seven centimeters dilated, and her midwife was called. Olivia did not look like she was in transition or active labor, but with this being her third child, I wondered. The midwife promptly came, checked her, and declared she was still four centimeters and 90 percent effaced. The nurse had made a mistake. The dilation is determined by inserting a couple of fingers inside the woman's vagina and ascertaining how many centimeters the cervix is open. It is not unusual that different people will have different opinions as to how much a woman is dilated, although this was a rather huge discrepancy. Later we found out that the nurse was still in training.

The news of such little progress had taken Olivia away from her serenity, she was confused and exhausted. The doctors wanted to induce labor by using Pitocin, but thankfully, her religion forbids the use of drugs going against the natural way of things unless it is an emergency. As an alternative, the midwife suggested castor oil. Castor oil is a potent laxative and has been used for many years to help induce labor. The theory is that the strong contraction of the peristaltic muscles, the intestines, stimulated by the laxative, will provoke the uterus to contract as well. That suggestion made her husband really happy. He had been very upset at the mistaken evaluation, and his spiritual leader had told him that castor oil was acceptable according to their religious literature.

After consulting with the midwife, I suggested they go home and take a nap and wait another twenty-four hours before they did anything. Being in labor and having diarrhea at the same time is just not a good thing. Olivia was very relieved and embraced the idea of going home to her own bed.

Saturday, at 5:00 a.m., I received another call from the doctor at the hospital. Olivia and her husband had just gotten to the hospital and she was now five centimeters dilated. The doctor explained, "They want you to come in right away." I joined them and we progressed for a while, waiting for the midwife to walk to the hospital.

When I walked into the room I noticed that Olivia was in an altered state, managing the contractions in a world of her own. In that world, she could only read my lips and could not understand anyone else's. She was "in the zone" and had opened the door only for me to join her. She was exhausted from the very long labor at home and had not slept for two days. She asked for an epidural. The midwife checked her and she was seven centimeters. I looked at her and told her she could make it if she wanted, but I would be glad to get whatever she needed. At 7:20, her bag of waters was ruptured by the midwife, and by 7:30 she began to hug her baby out (push).

During this phase, I noticed that every time she opened her eyes to read my lips and follow instructions to birth her baby she would lose concentration and couldn't push properly. That is when the Divine Spirit whispered in my ears a different way of communication with Olivia. I told her that I would squeeze her hand as long as she needed to push, and then release the hold when she needed to relax and breathe in. I also told her I would pat her fingers if we needed her to stop pushing and pant, in case the midwife needed to get the cord off the baby's neck. Olivia relaxed and closed her eyes holding tightly to my hand. We began riding the waves of labor again, this time her eyes closed, her concentration intact. The only contact with the outside world was my squeezing hand. After I quickly explained how I would communicate with Olivia, everyone went silent. The only sound came from her husband standing at her head, facing the wall behind her as he began chanting the sacred words in his prayer book.

She pushed for another forty-five minutes, and the baby's head came out. I patted her fingers and she began panting, while the midwife removed the twice-wrapped cord from around the baby's neck. Then back to hugging her baby out. At 8:28 a.m., a beautiful eight-pound, three-ounce baby girl graced this world.

This experience taught me how magical and private birth can really be without anyone needing to direct the mother to push this way or that and without the usual yelling that goes on at a birth in a hospital. This time, we were in a sacred space, surrounded by prayers—two women holding hands on a joyful and amazing journey.

THE POWER OF PRAYERS

Life will grant all your requests as long as you have faith. Do you know what you really want? You might answer, "Well, of course I know! I want to be happy, healthy, and more prosperous! What a silly question! Everyone wants that!" Yes, it is true. We all want all those things, but how do we ask for them? And more importantly, do we believe we deserve them?

CONSIDER THE LILIES OF THE FIELD, HOW THEY GROW; THEY TOIL NOT, NEITHER DO THEY SPIN. . . . IF GOD SO CLOTHE THE GRASS IN THE FIELD . . . SHALL HE NOT SO MUCH MORE CLOTHE YOU.

MATTHEW 6:28–31

When we pray, we often plead to our God the following way: "Please, God, I need money to pay this bill," or "Please, God, I want to feel better." What we are really expressing is our fears about a lack of money or health, and we buy into the concept that we are separate from God and that we live a life of limitation. As you recite this type of prayer, you may be wondering where this miracle is going to come from, or if you even deserve what you are asking for. When you say, "I want to feel better," you are concentrating on how bad you feel. When you focus on what you don't have, your energy is in the wrong place.

Have you thought about the exact thing that you want? Have you dreamed as big as you can? Do you really feel, deep inside, that you deserve it? Do you think your Higher Power loves you enough to be happy to give it to you?

The way we send out the message is as important as the message itself. If you ask to feel better, you are not really asking to be healed. If you are asking for some peace, you are not asking for complete peace. Today, try changing your prayers and act as if you have already received what you desire. "My God is the God of plenty and I now receive all that I desire or require, and more," or "Thank God for the peace that pervades my entire life right now," or "Thank you, God, for every day I feel healthier and wiser and blessed by your presence in my life."

God, the universe, and your mind work on faith. By faith, Abraham and Sarah had a child at the age of ninety. By faith, Moses parted the sea. By faith, Jesus raised Lazarus from the dead. They did not linger, they did not ask please, they forged forward by faith, and by faith, miracles manifested. Check inside yourself and see if the things you have been asking for in your prayers carry the faith that can and will make them come true. Know in your heart that you deserve them.

Prayer of Surrender

Father, I surrender myself into your hands; do with me what you will. Whatever you may do, I thank you. I am ready for all; I accept all. Let only your will be done in me, and in all your creatures—I wish no more than this. I know you will protect me and you will provide for me. You are my Father and I am safe within your arms.

Mother, I offer this child to you. Carry her today, care for her, love her, and nurture her. Carry me, love me, and nurture me, for today I will be the child in your sweet embrace. Today, I will treat myself as the child that is growing inside my womb. I will care for myself, I will love myself, I will nurture myself, and I will play, rejoice, laugh and say silly things, sing silly songs, hug all those I trust and love, and jump with joy. I will read a fairy tale to myself before I go to sleep, and I will sleep the slumber of a contented child, for I will know that tomorrow you will be there to hold me and love me all over again. And so it shall be.

MONTH
6

the right to see and to know the truth

I am aware of what I see, watch, and witness in my daily life. Vision and acceptance are intertwined with my intentions. I celebrate my inner vision and learn to use visualization to conquer and manage the waves of contractions. By seeing myself as a beautiful expression of the Divine, ready to see the beauty in others, I give life to an artist. I am fully Spirit, and it is my right to see and be seen as I truly am: a perfect expression of the Divine. I am grateful for my vision. I am thankful for my sight. I release these words into the cosmos. It is done, and so it is. Amen.

YOUR BABY NOW

Your baby is between twelve and fifteen inches long and weighs approximately two pounds. His eyes open and close, and his vocal cords are functioning. His lungs are filled with amniotic fluid, and he has started breathing motions. If you talk or sing, he can hear you. If you shine a bright light on your belly, he will be able to notice the change. Babies use their hands to shield their eyes. You will feel him pedaling and pushing his feet against your belly. You can play a tapping game with him: tap gently on your tummy, then wait a few minutes and he will tap back.

THE SIXTH CHAKRA

The sixth chakra is the energy center that governs the mind. Here we learn how to see and know the truth. This chakra is the seat of wisdom, vision, intuition, and our concepts of reality. As the baby discovers light and responds to it, his outer and inner sight are beginning to form. Your lesson this month will be to separate the mind from the spirit. The mind often gets in the way. We over-think, over-analyze, and over-process, inhibiting our natural intuition with our mind's constant chatter. Make sure that it is your inner vision that runs your life, rather than the vision of those around you. Beware also of not getting stuck in what you think your life should look like according to someone else's rules or expectations.

THE RIGHT TO SEE

Sight is, for most of us, the first filter through which we sift through our experiences. We often categorize, judge, and label people, places, and things based on what our eyes have seen. Labeling and judging is heavily influenced by our memories and the memories of primary caretakers. We now know that the baby has been accumulating our memories and is beginning to react and embrace our reactions to the environment. She is preparing herself for the kind of world we are portraying through our reactions, emotions, and state of being. Science explains this phenomenon: "It is now recognized that when the child is born, he is fully capable of experiencing almost all the emotions of adults. Newborns can express rage, jealousy, anger, love, and sadness. It turns out that both the mother and father are actually tailoring and shaping the child's physiology and behavior to fit into their world. If the parents find the world troubling, their child will be affected."[32] Often the world we experience is colored by the chatter that goes on in our minds. Instead of seeing things as they truly are we see the reflection of our own state of mind. For example two people can enter a room and, depending on their state of mind, have a completely different experience. One, who is happy about her life and how things are, can walk into the room and notice beautiful objects around the room and focus on the two people who smile at her. Another, who is burdened by constant judgment, will notice what is misplaced or wrong in the room and those people who seem angry, unhappy, or not to be trusted. It largely depends on the dialogue that goes on in our minds.

Once I realized how important it was to become conscious of the dialogue that happens in my mind, I conducted an experiment and went on a different kind of journey. I visited my mind.

My Mind

In a deep state of self-hypnosis, I visualized my mind as a big mansion, and as I looked around, I noticed that it was crowded with many people. A whole committee was living up there, including a judge, a worrier, a complainer, my mom and dad, my brother, and even the nun who was my first grade teacher. Each one had a room in my mind's mansion. All these people had permanently chosen quarters and set up camp. They burst in every time I needed to make a decision or when something happened to me. Then they held a meeting and argued about what I should do, what I should think, and how I should feel.

I recognized that I often became paralyzed while they were discussing *my* life and *my* future. After further analysis, I noticed that this group of people wasn't really improving the large mansion they had invaded. In fact, they were degrading it. They chimed in every chance they got, pronouncing that I should be ashamed of myself, dictating when I should be scared, and telling me when I should distrust my intuition or gut feelings. They had an opinion about every instance of my life and, at times, they even fought with one another. Some days, their fighting was so intense that I just couldn't get out of bed.

I decided to evict them all. That's right, "Out you go. Pack your stuff, and good riddance!" They didn't like that very much, but I put my foot down and made sure they all left the mansion inside my mind! It took some time and a bit of negotiating, but they finally left. I knew they'd probably want to come back because they really liked it there, so I resolved to change the locks of my mansion. I installed Self-Love as the security guard at the door to insure they couldn't return.

Once they had all departed, I looked around and saw that I had a huge, wonderful home inside my mind. As I opened its windows to let in the light and the fresh air, I began to plan how to redecorate and invite my new family. I decided to invite a nurturing and loving mother, a protective and wise father, a supportive and entertaining brother, and above all, a forever-loving Higher Power. Together we would rebuild that mansion. The windows would overlook the shores of trust, faith, and self-worth, and the ocean of serenity, peace, and harmony. By clearing my mind and ridding myself of all the chatter that no longer served me, I was able to create a new environment that allowed me to use unconditional love as the new paradigm through which I experience reality.

Once the filtering system has been taken care of, pay attention to the images you allow to enter your visual realm. Surround yourself with beautiful and serene images.

YOU ARE WHAT YOU WATCH

I recall my mother imparting the following wisdom to a pregnant friend of hers: "From now on, look only at smiling babies and always carry a beautiful rose." According to Italian superstition, an expectant mother should focus only on beautiful imagery. In fact, Italian lore goes as far as believing that if a pregnant woman looks at deformity during her state, she might risk giving her child a similar deformity. It is also believed that if a pregnant woman strongly craves a food and touches any part of her body during the height of the craving, the baby will have a birthmark in that spot. Italians are particularly worried about chocolate and wine cravings since birthmarks generally come in brown and purple shades. Several countries around the world have similar superstitions. In China, for example, the pregnant empress was forbidden to see anything but beauty. If anyone with any defect or lack of beauty was in her line of vision, they risked being killed. Although these are certainly old wives' tales, there just might be some message in them worth considering.

When we look at beautiful art or a horror film—or the news—we experience a series of emotions. Emotions are tied to our biochemistry, and every time we emote, our body produces hormones that either enhance or are detrimental to our health and well-being. Fear, anxiety, and terror cause an increase of the stress hormones adrenaline and cortisol. Watching a scary movie triggers the fight-or-flight response associated with adrenaline. Adrenaline steps up the heart rate, increases respiration, activates muscles by tensing them up, and promotes hyper-alertness. Cortisol, when it stays at high levels, automatically breaks down non-essential organs and tissues to maintain blood sugar and feed vital organs. Cortisol has been associated with aggression, depression, addiction, and pain. On the other hand, soothing or reassuring stimuli cause an increase in oxytocin, also known as the love hormone. We produce it naturally when we love, are loved, nurture another, give unconditionally, or engage in affectionate touch. This hormone not only induces emotional bonding, it is the key ingredient for labor and lactation. If love could be put in a pill, one of its ingredients would definitely be oxytocin.

THE PROPHET

Have you noticed how there is at least one type of altar in all homes? If you enter most homes around the world, regardless of religion and culture, they all have the same prophet as the centerpiece in their living room. The wealthier have one altar piece per room, and most people have spent more on this object than on any other individual item in their house. The prophet speaks to them, tells them how to feel, what to think, what to buy, what to like and dislike. It entertains them, makes them cry, keeps them current, and gives them information about the world. Most people spend an average of four and a half hours per day in front of the prophet, listening and learning, mesmerized by its power. In a crisis, people have been known to spend up to twenty hours in front of the prophet. Some have the prophet on just to keep them company even when they are doing other things around the house. You guessed it. The prophet is the television.

When I go to a client's house, I pay attention to their prophet. Is it on as I walk in? Do they turn it off as soon as I arrive, or does the woman nudge the husband to do it because I am there? When I visit them after the birth, I also notice if the mother is constantly in front of the tube as she is breastfeeding and resting with her baby. Then I ask, "How many hours of television do you think your child should watch, and starting at what age?" Inevitably I hear, "Oh we don't really want to be the kind of parents who put our child in front of the tube for hours. We'll let her watch very little." If you don't want your child watching a lot of television, you have to model that behavior yourself from the very beginning.

We teach by example, and some of the behaviors we freely exhibited before we were parents might need to be checked. This is a time to notice what you look at and what you watch each and every day, because it often determines your mood. People who constantly listen to the news have a tendency to be more irritable and pessimistic than those who do not. Those who watch soap operas have a tendency toward gossip, even if it is about the television stars. Be conscious when you turn on the tube. Why are you doing it and for how long? The more television you watch, the less you read, communicate with your partner, and use your imagination. The more you are hooked on a particular program, the more your child will learn the same behavior and the less time you'll spend with one another.

New research confirms that every hour an infant spends watching baby videos is associated with slower language development. According to the study, video-exposed babies score six to eight words less on a standardized vocabulary test than babies who are not exposed to videos.[33]

HOW WE SEE AND HOW WE ARE SEEN

Comparing can be an addictive behavior and may lead to sadness, anger, jealousy, and dissatisfaction. When we compare ourselves to others, we do a disservice to all. When we compare the progression of our pregnancy, or the development of our children with another, we shift the focus from loving what *is* to wishing for what *isn't*.

When you look at yourself and others with compassion, you will notice that everything and everyone is special. We all have a very important part in this universe, and we have all been given many lessons to teach and learn. Nothing is superfluous or unimportant or unnecessary. There are no mistakes for those who care to pay attention. When you find yourself spending time making comparisons, ask yourself the following questions: What am I to learn from this, or from this person? What am I to understand about this feeling I have of being less or more than someone?

Comparison stems from insecurity, insecurity fuels fear, and as we have learned, fear can harm us and our child. If you catch yourself comparing your pregnancy, doctor, body, or, once the baby is born, his or her development, use the three S's exercise: Stop, Shake it off, and Start over.

INNER VISION BIRTH PLAN

Nowadays, many women write a Birth Plan, an official document they give to their healthcare professionals, describing their desires for the upcoming labor and birth. In Southern California, many nurses ask for it and expect it, but in most hospitals around the country, we are far from such acceptance. Even though it's a good idea to put your desires down on paper, I've noticed that, depending on the tone of the Birth Plan, sometimes it can actually work against you. The document is at times mistaken as a declaration of mistrust in the people who will attend your birth. It can also limit instinctual, spur-of-the moment decisions, which might turn out to be more appropriate than a plan scripted several months before the event.

A Birth Plan can be seen as challenging by the medical staff, creating a defensive mindset. Most importantly, it can create a barrier to a deep, personal, and trusting relationship with those who will help you deliver your baby. I have seen nurses decide to "teach someone a lesson" by making sure that nothing in the Birth Plan was respected. In such a case, each obstacle to a part of the plan was presented as either a matter of "hospital policy" or as "too dangerous for this particular situation." What I often tell my clients is to work on going into the hospital with love pouring out of every fiber of their being and love for each individual who cares for them. I tell them to engage in friendship with the attending nurse by asking her about her own birth and children. If you show her respect, she'll be a lot more likely to want to help you fulfill your dream of having a natural, drug-free birth without medical intervention. I also suggest that if you're going to use a Birth Plan, make sure you add some personal information to it, such as a picture of your family and some short anecdotal phrases to describe yourself.

It's a good idea to spell out, on paper, what we would like to manifest, but it's best to approach this document as you would a love note.

Consider these excerpts from my clients' Birth Plans.

- I really have a phobia about a hospital setting; I get frightened easily when I don't understand what's going on. I would love to have a nurse who will help me understand all the procedures before they are performed.

- I can relax more easily when the lights are turned down, and I am frightened of needles. My husband and I have worked very hard to achieve a stress-free birth and I prefer to be able to move around during labor in order to manage my contractions. We prefer not to have an IV hooked up, but are willing to have a Heplock.[34] We trust you know what to do in case of an emergency.

- I have put a lot of effort into learning different techniques to use during labor to manage the contractions. I appreciate your help and suggestions on alternative methods of pain management, and I will certainly let you know if I want pain relief, but I would rather not be continually reminded about the drugs that are available. Please don't ask me to rate my pain from one to ten as it will distract me.

- Once our baby is born please help us bond with our child by keeping the conversation around us to a minimum, allowing mother and child to cuddle up skin to skin bundled up in warm blankets.

- We have been trying to get pregnant for a very long time, and are so happy we finally made it. We want to touch and hold our baby as soon as possible, and have even created a little song to sing to him immediately after birth. We feel very strongly about wanting to bond with our child and we prefer that all drugs like the eye ointment and the Vitamin K shot be administered two hours after the birth. If all has gone well, we want to avoid giving the baby a bath until later. Please evaluate our baby's Apgar[35] score while he is in our arms. Bathing, weighing, and measuring our child is not that important to us: we prefer holding, kissing, and having him suckle at mom's breast right away. We understand you have to follow procedure, but we ask that you allow us to enjoy skin to skin contact with our infant newborn as long as possible. We prefer that no pacifiers or bottle be given unless there is an emergency, and then only after you have discussed the situation with us and the pediatrician.

The more you humanize your desires and approach the hospital staff with friendly suggestions, the more you'll get what you want and need. I also encourage the family to attach a little gift basket to the plan for the nurses. This can help them taste the sweetness of your intentions as they read your Birth Plan.

Before you write your Birth Plan, identify your preferences and determine what remains to be clarified. You can find a Birth Plan questionnaire through your doula or on my Web site at www.joyinbirthing.com. Finally, it's always a good idea to show your Birth Plan to your practitioner and then ask him or her to sign it. This way, it will carry a lot more weight at the hospital.

THE RIGHT TO KNOW THE TRUTH

Some of the experiences we had as children might have been horrible, but if we're going to make a commitment to ourselves to live a conscious and happy life, we need to get rid of past resentments. Though you may feel righteous indignation for the people who hurt you, and it may be challenging to let go of the hurtful memories, doing so will free you from the hold they have on you. Sometimes what happens in our present life mirrors the lesson we still have to learn or the healing that still needs to take place. As we look at the truth of our relationships, we can see that other people are often mirrors reflecting an aspect of ourselves we need to pay attention to. Here's how my friend Elisabeth realized we attract the image and likeness of ourselves.

Elisabeth's Story: Looking in the Mirror

My friend Elisabeth decided to have a child on her own and called me to announce her decision. As we spoke she revealed her frustration, "I keep attracting men who are unable to commit; I call them the Pez boys, they might look different on the outside, but inside it's the same candy. I am not getting any younger, so I decided that I'm going to have a child on my own." I welcomed her choice and offered her a hypnotherapy session. Once under hypnosis, her righteous and willful persona relaxed, and she voiced some of the fears rooted beneath her decision. She was afraid of being too old with little time left to wait for "mister right," and "mister right now" was not interested in having a child. She wanted to be a mother, but was scared of having a baby on her own, and she was angry at the men in her life.

We focused on her original statement, "I keep attracting men who are unable to commit," and used the mirror technique, substituting "me" when we refer to another. For example: "I keep attracting me. I am not able to commit." As she pronounced this statement, she had one of those lightbulb moments. "Wow, I can't believe it, but this statement rings true, more so than the other," she observed. I suggested she write a list of complaints she had about her relationships and use the mirror exercise to shed some light into what she projected. Here's what she discovered:

- John can't express his feelings. He hardly ever tells me he loves me. = *I* can't express *my* feelings to John. *I* hardly ever tell *myself* I love *me*. I can't express my feelings to me.
- John isn't good with money. He is constantly worried

about his job and doesn't pay attention to me. = *I am not good with money. I am constantly worried about John and his finances, and I don't pay attention to me. I am constantly worried about me and my finances.*

- John is always looking to see if there is something better to do than to go out with me. = *I am always looking to see if there is something better than John, and something better than to go out with me. I'm always looking to see if there's something better than me.*

- John is always very distraught when I am depressed. He hates being with me unless I am in a good mood. = *I am always distraught when I am depressed and when John is depressed. I hate being with me unless I am in a good mood.*

The awareness that she was the one who was afraid of commitment and was attracting and manifesting herself through others allowed her to see the teaching the universe was bringing to her. Unless she became willing to commit to herself and be happy with herself, the universe would offer the lesson over and over again through the wrong relationships.

Elisabeth embarked on a mission of self-love and appreciation. She joined a twelve-step group, Co-Dependents Anonymous, and got a sponsor. She made the very first commitment in her life: to herself. Her affirmation was, "I am grateful for all the teachers and all the teaching that comes into my life. Today I am madly in love with me."

She still wanted to be a mother and used the Nine Basic Human Rights to prepare for parenting. She had been able to work through the first few chapters of *The Nine Basic Human Rights* workbook[36] until she got to the right to love and be loved. When asked to remember the first time she felt loved, she said that she was at a loss. She tried hard to go back and remember, but for some reason she just couldn't find a single moment in her past when she felt deeply loved. When asked to remember the good times associated with her childhood, she drew a blank. All she had chosen to keep in her immediate memory were the bad times, so her instinctual response was, "It was so bad, I can't recall anything good."

Elisabeth had experienced physical and emotional abuse from both her parents, one an alcoholic and the other a co-dependent. An army daughter, she had traveled all her life, changing schools and cities so often she felt she had no roots. With encouragement, she slowly began to recall little things that had given her some happiness and made her feel loved. She recalled a few episodes here and there: when her mother would take her to get ice cream on Sundays, or when her dad gave her first bicycle. She recalled summer vacations with her grandmother, time away that had given her some sense of stability. Slowly, she developed a list of happy memories. She set out to visualize those moments and recall as many details as possible, so that she could run a movie in her head that resembled a happy childhood. For years, she had chosen to hold onto and only remember the events that had made her suffer. She learned that with the help of her Higher Power, through prayer and meditation, she could switch the memories that linger in her present consciousness, and give over to God the ones that were hurtful.

After six months, she moved abroad and found a sperm donor. Nine months later, she gave birth to a beautiful son. "I had to create the man who'd want to live with me," she mused on the phone with me one day. Yet, kidding aside, she was happy about her decision and the work she had done on herself, knowing she could teach her child how to live consciously and love himself.

OBSERVE YOURSELF

Understanding what kind of person you are will help you to know what kind of labor activities will work for you. Observe what you do when you feel stressed out, nervous, anxious, or in pain. If as soon as you get a headache, you reach for the painkiller, you're likely to run for an epidural once you get to the hospital. The same goes for if, before you were pregnant, you quickly reached for the glass of wine or a cigarette or sugar. All those substances chemically alter your state so that you can numb your senses and escape what's at hand. However, since you became pregnant you've had to give up most of those substances; you know now that you can rely on alternatives to deal with whatever makes you feel sick, anxious, or uncomfortable. This is a good time to study yourself and notice the new coping mechanisms you've created for yourself and the positive ones that have worked for you through the years.

Are you someone who goes to the acupuncturist, homeopathic doctors, or chiropractor to relieve stress and tension? If so, continue to use this support system as it has been proven very helpful in achieving a natural childbirth. If you love to climb into a warm tub or isolate yourself in the shower, you'll enjoy the shower or tub during labor. If you are going to give birth at the hospital, make sure your partner brings a bathing suit so he can join you. If you are one of those who can't stay still, go on a walk as often as possible during labor, and alternate walks with rest, food, and water. If you like comfy clothes and are used to hugging blankets as you read a good book or listen to music, you'll want to put some thought into what to wear during labor and delivery. A hospital gown can throw you off center enough to go unconscious and tense up. Be sure to prepare the music you'll want to hear while in labor. If when managing pain, you prefer not to be touched or talked to, tell your partner and doula in advance. There's no need to cope with feelings of guilt simply because you feel they should partake in your journey. Witnessing a woman focused and in an altered state of bliss while in labor is an amazing experience no matter how the people around her participate in it.

I had a client who designed beautiful flash cards with powerful affirmations on them. She was a visual person and wanted to make sure there was some sort of art she could focus on during labor. After waiting nearly two weeks past her due date, her doctor decided she needed to be induced. Even though she had hoped to labor naturally, she had prepared herself. During the toughest Pitocin-laced labor contractions, she asked her husband to show her the flash cards. She would lose herself in the images and repeat the affirmations written on the cards. She managed the contractions well without an epidural and delivered a sweet baby girl. The experience was so amazing for her, she later decided to become a doula.

Learning what works for you when you are in pain or during stress is very important. Visualizing how you'd like the birthing environment to be will help you make the necessary preparations.

KNOWING WHAT IS RIGHT FOR YOU

Loyalty, honor, and justice are tribal traits. When taken to their extreme, they can cause great pain and suffering. At times, we are extremely loyal, remaining in harmful situations too long, and we often allow our tribal beliefs to stand in the way of our better judgment. Doctors are sometime seen as gods in our society. We believe they can do no wrong, especially if we don't feel we have the same amount of schooling under our belt. I see this regularly with my clients.

No matter how much information they have gathered to understand each and every procedure, once at the hospital, they forsake their own instincts and embrace their doctor's opinion without question. Except in an emergency, birth is not a medical event. Each one of us has an innate ability to know what is right for our own body and our child. We need to collaborate with our caretakers, not let them take over our care.

I met a woman at one of my lectures who complained about her doctor: "He makes me cry every time I see him. When I told him I didn't want to have an epidural, he told me I was crazy. He treats me like a little girl." I asked her if she would go back to a hairdresser after a terrible haircut. "Of course not," she responded. "Then why go back to the same doctor?" I exclaimed, trying to keep composure. "After all, we live in Los Angeles and there are thousands of doctors to choose from who are just as qualified." She told me she felt she should be loyal to him since he had seen her since the beginning of her pregnancy. I suggested she let her intuition advise her and ask her baby directly for his input. As I embraced her to say goodbye, I reminded her that everything would work out and that she had all the knowledge she needed to be the best mom for this particular baby, or he would not have chosen her.

This was an intelligent woman, one who had made many important decisions in her career, one who could negotiate great deals for her clients. What had happened? Why did she lose her self-esteem and confidence when confronted by her doctor? Giving birth and parenting are two of the most important jobs a woman will ever have, yet no one has bothered teaching us the basics. In the past, there was the village, and we learned by watching other women, our mothers, cousins, aunts, or sisters. We witnessed some births and saw women breastfeed their babies. We knew it was a natural process. We learned the tricks and the joys, and we gained confidence. Today, we are all little islands. Most of my clients have never even held a newborn, let alone seen one breastfed, changed, bathed, or birthed. Thus, we abdicate all powers to our provider. But should we? When it comes to wanting a natural birth, it's not important to ask our doctor's opinion about the alternative ways we choose to give birth, but we do need to ask for their support. Doctors are there to give us a medical opinion and we are very grateful for that. Keep in mind, though, that how you are going to have your baby—whether you choose to do it without medication or with the help of a doula, whether you choose to deliver squatting or on all fours—those are your decisions and no one else's.

I met that same woman after she had her baby. She told me that she had finally gotten the courage to change doctors, she had met a group of midwives that operated out of a hospital and she felt so happy with them after the initial visit it turned out it had not been so hard after all to let her doctor go. That had been the best decision she had ever made. You could see the love in her eyes, self-love and appreciation for standing up for herself.

It is your right to have the birthing experience you desire. Get informed, go to classes, get a doula, bring your village, find a woman who has gone through the kind of birthing experience you would like to have and speak to her. Don't stay in any harmful situations out of loyalty to anyone. Your loyalty should reside only with yourself and the well-being of your child.

PREPARE YOUR BIRTHING IMAGERY AND POWER WORDS

In his book *Mind Over Labor,* Carl Jones goes to great length to explain how the mind influences childbirth in a remarkable way, and how using mental imagery can alter the course of labor.[37]

In hypnosis, we use imagery and power words to maintain a connection with the laboring woman during the last few hours leading to a birth. Often at this stage in her labor, she enters an altered state of consciousness and loses connection with the outside world.

You may recall Susan's experience walking into the hospital while in active labor. She said, "I wasn't really there. I didn't look at anyone or anything. I hung onto my doula while she talked to people. It wasn't that I was upset or anything, I literally just had to focus on one thing: what was happening inside of me. The tremendous earthquakes that were shaking my core. Moving my center. It took all my focus. I heard everything that was going on around me, but my sight went. I didn't really take in the hospital. I had been worried about the clinical atmosphere of the hospital. I shouldn't have been. I was consumed by my internal world. Nothing like that made a dent on my inner events."

Justine writes of her experience: "They asked me if I wanted a mirror and I said, 'No, I'm way too busy for a mirror!' I didn't need one anyway, because I was literally having an out-of-body experience. I could see myself from the ceiling on the other side of the room, from over the doctor's shoulder."

I recall that with my own second child, when my midwife told me I had to dilate two more centimeters before I could push, I closed my eyes and imagined two little hands stretching my cervix over the baby's head. Within minutes, I was ready to hug my baby out.

Often, when a woman is stuck at a particular dilation, simply repeating, "open, open, open," will create the needed effect. It really helps when you familiarize yourself with the body parts involved in labor so that you can recall them and make them work for you.

KNOWING THE TRUTH

By now we know that in order to be free we have to let go of those things, people, and places that no longer serve us. And as we go through the letting go process, we discover that some things are harder to let go of than others. In my own self-discovery, I realized that no matter how hard I tried, I could not let go of certain people or events in my life. So instead of focusing on what I had to let go of, I began looking at *why* I didn't want to let go. As I had my daily conversation with God, I realized that discarding has been a point of great resistance in my life. I didn't want to let go of the memories, good or bad. I did not want to let go of my parents or my past lovers, even when the memories involved hurt and abuse. Being uprooted from my own country, I felt that those memories, hurtful or not, were my roots, and I feared that without them I would float at the whim of the wind. Hanging on seemed necessary for survival; it was the mechanism I used to fight loneliness. I learned this lesson as I went through a painful breakup.

Hanging onto the Wrong Truth

At the end of yet another intimate relationship, I found myself shipwrecked. I had been with this man for a short five months, and aside from three amazing weeks during the honeymoon period, I had already questioned the relationship and our compatibility. So when, after a brief fight over the telephone, I heard him say, "You know, when we talk, you don't seem to understand sh . . . t! I better go my way and you go yours," I swallowed hard and said "OK." I figured he would get over it and call me back. After all, he always called me twice a day, and we had survived prior disagreements. Days passed, and finally I called and left a message. No response from him. After a few more days, I wrote an e-mail, but still heard nothing back from him. A tsunami washed over me, and I began to feel a pain that was overwhelming.

I couldn't stop crying and my stomach hurt deeply as I asked myself, "Will I ever hear from him again?" I knew that this pain was way too much to be about just this relationship, so in tears I went to work. In my journal, I wrote answers to the following questions: What does this remind me of? What is my part in it?

I noticed a pattern: more than one man in my life had disappeared without a word, which has always been my worst nightmare. As I decided to investigate even deeper, I was overcome by a wall of grief and pain. As the pain intensified and I started to feel dizzy, I knew this was going to be a big revelation. I closed my eyes and allowed my inner vision to guide me into the past. I was able to look at myself in the present and saw that I was crying, repeating to myself and anyone who cared to hear it, "I just can't believe he won't talk to me again. After telling me he cared for me so much and so many times." Finally, I fell into a fitful slumber and saw myself in a little plastic crib, alone in a hospital nursery, feeling very similar emotions: "Ma è la mia mamma, perché non viene, perché non mi vuole bene?" ("But she is my mommy, why isn't she coming, why doesn't she love me?") I was feeling a pain that did not belong to this present moment, or to this relationship. What I was experiencing was ancient and very deeply rooted.

As I mentioned earlier, my mom had gone through so much pain during her labor that she did not see me for a couple of days after the birth, and even as an infant I had drawn a lifelong conclusion: I don't deserve to be alive, my mom has abandoned me, I am unlovable.

That statement shed light on the recurring fear of abandonment that had colored my relationships for many years. I recreated the same scenario over and over again with men so that I could attempt to heal my past vicariously through them. Once I came out of the self-hypnotic state, I looked at my relationship and noticed that I had created many of the circumstances, not only for this man, but for many of my relationships, where the best thing for them to do was to disappear from me.

I was the architect of it all, and that was an agonizing realization. My next question was to the heavens: "Now that I know, now what? This hurts, dear God. What do you want me to learn?"

I had prayed for a relationship to come into my life and had been so pleased that this man, who was Italian and spoke Italian, seemed to be instrumental in some of my healing. While with him, I had mended my relationship with my brother, and I had discovered the deep-seated need I had to heal my relationship with my Higher Power, specifically speaking my first language. When in conversations, I'd spoken the word *Dio*, Italian for God, and noticed that the word had a lot of baggage attached to it from my school days with the nuns. It had left a residue in my soul that needed to be cleared. Speaking Italian every day with this man and talking to him about my spirituality had helped me mend my relationship with my Higher Power in my own language. I had so much to be thankful for. Yet, now I had been abandoned all over again and had once more manifested my worse nightmare. I was far from understanding the reason I had to feel this much pain. So I went deeper . . .

Here is what I realized. Hanging on to the hurt of what happened in the past and what was happening in the present was only detrimental to my well-being. I became grateful for the failed relationship, because it offered me a chance to heal the past. Every day for the next few weeks, I consciously went back to that hospital nursery and talked to the child who felt abandoned. I reassured her of my love for her now and forever more. I showed her the bright and beautiful future she had ahead of her so I could instill hope in her little heart. I also visited my mom in her hospital bed when she was lost, alone, and in pain. I embraced her and told her about the love I would feel for her for the rest of my life. I reassured her that I knew it was not her fault, that there would be no blame, but only love flowing between us. I told her that now I understand that I cannot be abandoned unless I abandon myself.

If we want to find our pathway to healing, it is better to hurt and remember than to hurt and *not* remember. It is said our brain cannot distinguish between the past, the present, and the future, and that any message that is given to our subconscious mind for a minimum of thirty days will eventually become a reality in our consciousness.

The more we fight and resist our life history, the more it will persist. Even memories fight for their survival, and so do the behaviors we have learned in order to cope with those memories. The habits of self-judgment and self-abuse have a life of their own and struggle to survive. When we look at ourselves with love and know that any particular behavior we still implement was created for our own survival, put in place by a scared little girl, we can dissipate its strength. Infusing our past with love is the answer, not discarding the past, denying it, or ignoring it. All of it is perfect. God has a great design for our lives, the Divine is infallible, and there are no mistakes. All that has befallen is exactly what was supposed to happen. Life is, has been, and will be perfect as long as we are simply willing to love it all.

VISIONING: A MEDITATION

Take a deep breath in, and as you listen to your breath, you are going to go deeper and deeper into a state of total relaxation. That's it. Inhale deeply all the way into your belly; see your child feel the breath of fresh air coming from you. With each exhale, let all the stress and tension out. Take another deep breath and let all your thoughts pass through your mind.

Totally and completely relax all the muscles of your body, from the tips of your toes up through the trunk of your body. Take another deep breath and feel the energy spiraling up your spine, relaxing all your tiny muscles up your back and between your shoulder blades and your shoulders. Now pull the energy up to your throat, swallow once hard, then relax all the muscles in your face—around your mouth, your eyes, your ears, your forehead—and then all around your head.

Now imagine your life as if it were a tapestry. Consider the many stitches, all the different colored threads, the big and little knots. Feel the texture of these threads. Acknowledge all the work that went into creating this intricate tapestry.

Look at your tapestry from a distance. Observe the patterns. Yes, allow that smile on your face. Now admire your beautiful patterns. Honor all that has come, all that is, and all that is yet to come. Appreciate the complexity of some of your patterns. Muse at the simplicity of some earlier ones. Notice the holes in your tapestry, then look at the patches you have created to cover those holes. Some of those patches were placed there by you when you were a little child. You did your best not to interrupt the Divine weaving.

Recognize the effort your child-self put into creating those patches. Some of them were essential to your survival. Some may look funny to you right now. Some may not be as perfect as you want them to be. You didn't even know that some of these patches existed. Do not be critical of the loud colors or the funny stitches you see. You did the best job you could do at that particular time. Love all your little and big patterns and patches.

You have been in charge of creating your own tapestry all along. Today, you can weave in threads of self-love and compassion, Divine inspiration and humility. You can create a new pattern. You can fill in the holes with acceptance and forgiveness.

Celebrate, for you are a disciple of the Master Weaver. You can choose the colors, the design, and the direction of your new patterns. There are no mistakes in your tapestry; it is a Divine work of art.

Now You Know

Now you know that everything you do is sacred. Now you know that there are no bad people, places, or things, just teachers and lessons. Now you know that each teacher and lesson is invaluable. God has placed them on your path because She loves you very much. Now you know that good and bad and right and wrong are only a figment of your imagination. Now you know that you are the Divine child brought to give life and fulfill your destiny. Now you know that there are no mistakes in the Divine mind. Now you know that love is the key that opens all doors. Nothing that is asked in earnest can be denied.

As you wake up each morning, ask God for your heart's desire. Quiet the mind and listen to Her response. Trust and let Her guide you. Now you know that your changing body is radiant and beautiful.

You are able and willing to give your unborn child everything she needs to grow and be healthy. Now you know that everything you do is sacred.

Now you know.

MONTH

7

the right to consciousness

I channel the power of consciousness and enrich my life. I open myself to the messages I receive. I have the necessary information in order to achieve my goal of a natural and drug-free birth. I manifest the perfect team to help during labor and the postpartum phase. I see the light of God within each and every person that will participate in my birthing experience. I recognize that being conscious in every aspect of my life is powerful, and I harness this power for my own good. I strike a partnership with the Divine and teach my child how it's done; I cradle in my womb and give birth to my best teacher. Grateful for all this and much more, I simply let it be. And so it is. Amen.

YOUR BABY NOW

Your baby's lungs and digestive tract are almost fully developed. By now, your baby weighs about two and a quarter pounds and is about fifteen inches long. Her body is well formed. Your baby is continuing to grow and develop. The lanugo[38] is starting to disappear from her face. She can now hear the outside world quite well over the sound of your heartbeat. She exercises by kicking and stretching. She can also make grasping motions and likes to suck her thumb. She will even move in rhythm to music. Her lungs are still growing and are not yet mature. Patterns of your baby's brain waves appear like a full-term newborn.

THE SEVENTH CHAKRA

The seventh chakra, also called crown chakra, is about living consciously. It integrates all the chakras belonging to the human sphere, one through seven. It is often represented in Eastern art by a 1000-petaled lotus, symbolizing the entry point of Divine energy. In the same way that the cervix opens up during an orgasm for the sperm to impregnate the egg, the crown chakra represents the celestial cervix through which the Divine descends upon us during labor. It is the portal that connects us with God. In meditation, when the energy is raised up to seventh chakra, the illusion of individual self is dissolved. We become one with the cosmic principles that govern the entire universe within the body. During procreation the creative force journeys upward towards the divine and life is created. Then, and only in mothers, the eighth and ninth chakras are activated and the divine descends into the woman's body and becomes incarnate through her baby.

Whatever we have understood intellectually and intuitively up to this point will reach a whole new level of comprehension when the seventh chakra is working at full capacity. During the seventh month of gestation, the baby's brain is fully functioning and exhibiting rapid growth and development. It also has the ability to organize information.[39] The baby is now going from simply gathering knowledge to becoming conscious of itself. During the seventh month of pregnancy, we must learn to integrate our physical, emotional, and mental life into one fully conscious experience. Thus, we can open up our whole being to the power and presence of God. We are no longer victims of circumstance and we realize and teach our child the responsibility that goes with living in full awareness.

THE RIGHT TO CONSCIOUSNESS

Full consciousness comes with a price. You have relied on your five senses and your intellect to create reasonable expectations in your life. Your senses, combined with your acquired knowledge, gave you the illusion of being in control. However, now that you have been given a glimpse of a different path on your journey toward a painless childbirth, you'll come to realize that the illusion of control only creates further tension. Willingness is key; the only path to a painless childbirth is one of surrender and trust in the natural process.

Birth is unpredictable, but with all our wits about us, we can make informed decisions, talk to our body to gather more strength when it's needed, move around to facilitate the baby's descent, and be present and conscious when our little one joins us in this world. Our desire to be in control is only another form of resistance. It may not always be easy, but the beauty of living a conscious life is that it will allow you to reach higher peaks of happiness. As we recognize our power as a creator, we are consciously creating the life we choose, and learning to live and grow in joy.

Your serenity and sense of self will be so strong, nothing will stand in your way, and as a mother you will be a pillar of knowledge and love to your child. Your teaching motto will be: do as I do. When you are living consciously, what you choose to focus your energy upon will grow.

Conscious living becomes easy when we are happy, satisfied, and accept the truth that the world around us is a peaceful one. This sense of peace is thrown into imbalance only when we are angry, hungry, sick, or tired.

CONSCIOUS LABOR

When you're angry, hungry, sick, or tired, you're more likely to indulge in behaviors you will later regret. Consider how many times you have found yourself saying, "I can't believe I said that," or "I can't believe I did that." If you look back at those inopportune moments, you'll invariably find that what you regret is something you did while you were angry, hungry, sick, or tired.

When we experience these feelings our mature conscious-self is weakened, and our unconscious-self steps forward. The unconscious-self is often childlike because its responses are based on coping mechanisms, beliefs, attitudes, and behaviors that were created when we were children. When faced with a challenge, we learned to react a certain way in order to survive, to be loved, or to be liked and accepted. Extra vigilance is required of us when we're weakened by anger, hunger, sickness, or fatigue, because each of these challenges will come up during labor and delivery. By discovering what our unconscious and automatic responses are to these sensations, we can better prepare for dealing with them consciously during labor.

During labor, the intensity of the contractions and the feeling of being overwhelmed may arouse anger within you.

You may experience hunger if you go to a hospital where laboring women are not allowed to eat, and you might have the impression that you're sick, given the hospital setting, the intensity of the waves, and the overall unfamiliarity of the situation. And, of course, you'll be tired because labor is a lot of work!

ANGER

Anger happens when we think that things aren't going our way, when we think that our needs and desires aren't being met, when we concern ourselves with what others think of us, or when we worry that God is giving us something we cannot handle. The intensity of our feelings is proportionally related to our fears about what others think of us and how important it is for us to be right. When we lash out in anger, our reactions almost always stem from fear. Afraid of abandonment, we scream at a lover when we imagine the faintest possibility that he will leave us, or that he does not care about us as much as we care about him. Fearing that we are not good enough, we read into others' words what we fear they truly think of us, and in fact, what we truly think of ourselves. We fear our choices are not right, thus anyone who contradicts us reminds us of our own doubt, and we engage in screaming matches to prove them wrong. We fear we'll lose the respect of others if we are not right, and so we fight fiercely for our need to be right. We fear we are not capable of doing something, and so we fight and belittle others who mirror our self-perceived incompetence. As we react to all that we see, say, hear, know, want, do, think, and emote, an entire chemistry is unleashed.

When we are angry, our body tightens, our muscles contract, some of us begin trembling, and we become short of breath. Hormones are released in our bloodstream and rush through our vascular system's highway to reach every cell in our body and our baby's body, communicating a message of stress and resistance. These are all conditions that prevent us from relaxing and having a painless childbirth.

To interrupt these negative, established patterns of self-defeating behavior and to train ourselves to live more consciously, it's important to identify the roots of our fears and the agreements we have made with ourselves about how to behave in moments of distress. If you look at your pattern of reactions that follow feelings of anger and where they come from, you can empower yourself to heal and redirect them while in labor.

Carmen's Story

Carmen was walking one day at the beach, contemplating whether to have a homebirth or a hospital birth. Since I take my dogs to the beach every day, our paths crossed. I was on the telephone with a colleague, recounting the latest birthing experience I witnessed. After my telephone conversation ended, Carmen approached me. "Excuse me," she inquired, "I couldn't help but hearing that you're somehow involved in the birthing industry. Are you a midwife?" After I explained to her what I do, she said, "I can't believe the coincidence! Here I am asking God to send me a sign so that I can make up my mind about home or hospital birth, and as soon as I finish my request, I meet you!"

We talked at length about the pros and cons of both choices, and I asked her to look inside herself and ask which one made her feel more comfortable and happy. She decided that she wanted a homebirth and I suggested a few midwives she could interview. Once the midwife was chosen, Carmen wanted to do some hypnotherapy to rid herself of the fear attached to her decision about a homebirth.

During the hypnosis sessions, we made some serious discoveries. Carmen was raised by a very controlling mother and at an early age was molested by a neighbor. These two experiences were the roots of her fears and anger. Carmen, as a little girl, had come to the conclusion that she did not deserve to have her desires fulfilled. After having heard so often as a child, "You don't know what you're doing," she totally embraced that belief. When asked the question, "How does that belief manifest itself in the decisions you make on a daily basis?" she responded that she constantly questioned her own judgment and would have long, exhausting fights with herself about every important decision. Furthermore, she was often very angry at her husband, who never seemed to do the "right" thing.

To heal such a core belief, we did two things. First, we went through the Feelings Inventory Exercise, and from the writing she discovered that her core belief about herself, ever since she was a little girl, was that she was a helpless person who didn't deserve to be happy. Her coping mechanism was to become angry every time she felt helpless or out of control. She also had a lot of anger toward her husband, whose love she couldn't quite justify in her child-self's mind. We developed an affirmation that she would repeat to herself twice a day: "I am capable of making decisions about my well-being and I deserve to be happy. I am lovable."

Once this mantra was in place, we proceeded with the next part of the healing process: we had to tackle the experience of being molested.[40] Using hypnosis, we went back to the first moment she felt she was helpless. In her case it was when the molestation began, and we brought the adult Carmen into the picture. Carmen now stood between her child-self and the perpetrating neighbor and demanded that he stop what he was doing and never do it again. I allowed her to find her own words to confront him. I coached her to tell him what she wanted to tell him without anger, but with a firm and resolute voice. I told her not to explain much to him, but to state her desires in a short sentence. I also suggested she listen for any response he might have. Surprisingly enough, he had quite a few. So she repeated several times, "I will no longer accept this. Stop and go away!" until he disappeared. Then I asked her to turn around and face her child-self. Adult Carmen went down on her knees and told her child-self that she would be with her from now on and that she would protect her. She also asked for a hug and promised never to abandon her. Tears were streaming down her face. She had worked on this issue for years with a therapist, but had never gone back to that very moment in time when it all began. By visualizing the incident and bringing her adult-self into the memory, she was able to change that memory. The healing and boundaries that her adult-self had effected within the re-visitation would now permanently be part of her memory.

When we came back to the present time, still under hypnosis, we visualized her fears of the homebirth as lit candles. We then asked the little Carmen to run up to the candles and blow her fears out.

The healing had begun! Carmen had a swift and lovely homebirth. She was very quiet and focused inward during the entire labor. She squatted for just a few minutes and her baby boy was born into her husband's hands.

A few weeks after the birth, I received a frantic phone call from her, "I'm very dizzy and my head is spinning. I need to get to the homeopathic pharmacy to get some remedies, but I'm afraid to drive and my husband won't help." I offered to drive her, and from the conversation we had on the way, I discovered that she had just had a big fight with her husband. Anger had once again unbalanced her, and regardless of whether it was justified or not, the power of the emotion was enough to create dizziness, which is a typical symptom of imbalance in the seventh chakra. After the babymoon,[41] her husband had to go back to work and a strong feeling of helplessness had engulfed her. Not believing she could do it all alone, take care of the child and herself, she resorted to her old way of coping: getting angry at her husband. Since she had done the workbook on the Nine Basic Human Rights, I suggested she use the three S's exercise—stop, shake it off, and start over—every time she felt anger bubbling up inside. I reminded her that even though she had experienced the natural, drug-free, and painless childbirth she had desired, she needed to continue her commitment to conscious living.

HUNGER

Let us examine the hospital policy of "nothing by mouth," also called NPO. NPO was an intervention created to deal with general anesthesia. In the old days, general anesthesia was administered via a mask. If a woman laboring on her back threw up into the mask, she ran a substantial risk of choking.

In the article, "Nutrition and Position In Labor," C. Johnson concludes: "No time interval between the last meal and the onset of labor guarantees a stomach volume of less than 100 ml." In other words, a laboring woman could fast for the entire duration of her labor, yet her stomach might nevertheless contain sufficient material to fatally choke her, should she throw up while lying down.[42] Ketosis is an abnormal increase in chemicals that your body produces when, after it has used up its available store of glycogen (blood sugar), it turns to burning fat. The 1999 World Health Organization report titled *Care in Normal Birth* states that ketosis is an unfavorable practice for both mother and fetus and can be prevented by offering the mother "light meals" during labor. The hospital has translated this into the solution of clear broths full of salt, and Jell-o full of sugar. Vegetarians can't have either one, for they both are derived from animal products. Inadequate consumption of complex carbohydrates results in low blood sugar, which produces less effective, and sometimes painful, uterine contractions. Less effective contractions slow labor and may lead to the diagnosis of "failure to progress," significantly increasing the chances of a Cesarean section.

I often tell my clients who have chosen a hospital birth that they need not go into detail with the nurses, explaining reasons behind the specific requests in their Birth Plan. All they have to do is present their Birth Plan with those requests signed by the doctor and ask for the nurse's support. So, to an insistent nurse who wants to place an IV on a laboring woman that supposedly brings life-saving "nutrients" to the depleted maternal bloodstream simply because it's hospital procedure, even though the Birth Plan states she prefers a Heplock, I suggest my client says, "No, thank you." There is no need to explain why, no need to get angry at the nurse.

My suggestion is to eat a good, hearty meal at the onset of your labor. Follow that with small meals throughout, such as avocadoes, tomatoes, lettuce, tahini, apples, nuts, energy bars, and protein drinks. These foods keep the laboring mother's blood sugar at a healthy level. Discuss this with your care provider and see if you can get her to allow you food as long as you are not medicated. When laboring at home, you can eat to your heart's content.

SICKNESS

Of course you are not sick! You're having a baby, and the experience, while intense, is not unnatural. During labor, two things often happen: First, strong sensations or contractions are very unfamiliar, and their intensity resembles something you've previously experienced only when sick. Second, you unconsciously believe that one only goes to the hospital when something is seriously wrong. Often, in the midst of active labor, clients give me a look that says, "What's wrong with me? This is intense!" That's when I remind them that this is what it feels like when the baby is working hard to come into this world. Then I encourage them to concentrate on the time *between* contractions.

Managing the waves of contractions one minute at a time, and focusing on the time in between when you experience the absence of painful sensations, is the key to fighting this feeling of disease. Prepare yourself to stay in the moment, and do not anticipate the next contraction. Manage one at a time and revel in the time in between. Illness does not permit such breaks! If you are birthing at home, keep reminding yourself that you're having a baby by visiting the nursery, looking at your baby's clothes, and fantasizing about holding your baby in your arms. Often, I suggest that the mother ask her unborn child what is his favorite color and whether he wants a special object, drink, or food during his entrance. This will become a great reminder to the mother that the baby is working as hard as she is in this process, and she becomes the adult encouraging the baby.

If you are going to a hospital, make sure you walk yourself to the labor and delivery ward. Decline, firmly but gently, the wheelchairs offered and, if you can, decline the hospital gown. Instead, use a loose T-shirt or nightgown that you can easily raise above your belly and that allows for easy access to your breasts. A hospital gown can be interpreted by your unconscious mind as proof that you have become a patient, as opposed to being a client who has chosen to avail herself of the hospital's birthing facility. Once in the room, lower the lights, put some soothing music on, and tell the staff that you want to walk and move around as much as possible, as long as everything is OK. The staff will want to check the baby's heartbeat, but all you really need is occasional monitoring. Make sure that you can take a bath or a shower, as you would at home. The gentle rolling of the water on your belly or back will definitely help you relax.

FATIGUE

Babies simply love to begin their journeys at night. In fact, they often choose to start their journey in the middle of the night, waking up the mother and making it difficult for her to go back to sleep. Labor often starts at night because you are finally totally relaxed and the body figures that it's a good time to start working. Total relaxation is the sure way to a gentler, painless childbirth. Alas, when we feel an intense sensation, our body goes into fight-or-flight mode and we tense every muscle. This tension prevents the uterus from having the space it needs to gently contract and, as I call it, "hug your baby all the way out!"

Since labor so often starts in the middle of the night, it is imperative that you talk to your care provider about ways you can relax. Ask their opinion about you having a single glass of wine. You should not have had any for nine months, so one glass will do the job at the onset of labor without any negative side effects. I know the mention of wine for a pregnant woman is considered taboo. Why it is OK to go to the hospital and have an opiate injected directly into our spine during labor, but alcohol is verboten, I'll leave you to evaluate. Other ways to relax and go back to sleep include: a soothing massage, a self-hypnosis tape, a warm bath, a cup of hot milk and honey, or an antihistamine often given to pregnant women to control itching, and known to cause drowsiness. In other words, be prepared with a bag of tricks to help you go back to sleep. If you cannot go back to sleep, then you might as well go on a walk (please don't do this alone and make sure it's in a very safe place), get on the treadmill, or make yourself a significant night snack. In Italy, we call it "spaghetti a mezzanotte" or "midnight spaghetti." Turn the music on and dance, but commit to taking a nap during the day before you leave for the hospital, if that's where you're going.

There are four main activities I suggest my clients rotate during labor: rest, eat and drink, walk, and take a bath or a shower. And of course, call your doula to let her know you are in labor so she can get prepared!

By observing the reactions you commonly have when you're angry, hungry, sick, or tired, you can learn to manage each state and be prepared for your labor and delivery. All these conditions are likely to shut down your recognition of what's really happening: you are simply having a baby. Those conditions or states trigger the unconscious mind, causing panic, tension, and stress. No matter how prepared you are, no matter how much you have visualized your desired outcome, know that your endurance has the potential to weaken under the intensity of the contractions. You can prepare yourself for these unpleasant moments by learning more about yourself and your reactions when in crisis.

CONSCIOUS CO-CREATION WITH YOUR CARE PROVIDER

Knowledge is power. Asking the right questions puts you in charge of your own well-being. Write down your questions before your appointment with your doctor or midwife. Go and visit the birthing place; familiarize yourself with the environment and make sure the people who work there will respect your personal preferences. Visit their nursery and talk to the visitors and families who are there. When a relative is hanging around waiting for a baby to be born, or cooing at a baby through the nursery window, they're eager to talk. Remember, you can change hospitals and doctors as many times as you need to, until you find what and whom you want. Don't be afraid. The following are seven questions you should ask your care provider in their office or while you are in the hospital before any procedure is performed:

1. Is this an emergency, or do we have time to talk?
2. What are the benefits of doing this?
3. What are the risks?
4. If we do this, what other procedures or treatments might I end up needing as a result?
5. What else can you suggest we try first or instead?
6. What would happen if we waited an hour or two (or a day or two, or a week or two, etc.) before doing it?
7. What would happen if we didn't do it at all?

Learn these questions by heart; they should be asked before any procedure, for the rest of your life. We live in intervention-happy times. Our care providers have sworn they will do anything they can to take our pain away, even before they figure out whether the pain is there for a "good" reason. Knowledge is power.

UNDERSTANDING EPIDURALS

A client once told me that she wanted an epidural as soon as she entered the hospital. She wanted to know what to expect and was convinced that if part of her lower body was numb, her brain would function fully and she would be able to be in charge. She had seen women who seemed out of control while in labor and she certainly didn't want to make a fool of herself. I told her that when you have an epidural, your entire body is numbed, your mind gets fuzzy, and you often need to go to sleep. It's a very powerful drug that affects both your body and brain. Furthermore, as soon as you have an epidural, the doors of medical intervention are pushed open, as there is no telling how your body and your child will react to it, what other procedures you might need, or what the outcome of your delivery will be. Thus, if the total abdication of control is what you seek, an epidural will do the job.

IF YOU ARE GOING TO HAVE AN EPIDURAL, HERE ARE THE FACTS

You will need an IV to be inserted prior to receiving the epidural. You will be confined to the bed, incapacitated from the waist down. You will lie in a supine position, and unless you have a very good nurse, you will not be moved very much, which will make the descent of your baby very difficult.

Studies have shown that there is an increased chance of a Cesarean birth instead of a vaginal birth when a woman is under the influence of an epidural.

You will need a urinary catheter because you will not be able to urinate on your own with the epidural. A catheter may increase your chances of a bladder infection or urinary tract infection, requiring antibiotics, which may cause you to have a yeast infection and cause the baby to have thrush.[43]

Drugs will increase the possibility of a vacuum forceps delivery if you are not able to effectively push the baby out, and they may increase the chance of an episiotomy because the IV may cause the perineum to become engorged and therefore prevent it from stretching to allow the baby to deliver easily.

Most of the time, an epidural will severely restrict the position in which you can push. If injected too high in the spine, the mother may feel like she can't breathe.

There are several potential allergic reactions. Some women have suffered consequences for years after the administration of an epidural.

Some studies indicate that inadvertent epidural punctures occur in 1.6–1.8 percent of women; 23 percent of these women experience an onset of chronic symptoms including headache, migraine, or neckache, starting within three months after childbirth and lasting from nine weeks to more than eight years. Thorp Mayberry states that these headaches can be severe enough to temporarily interfere with women's normal activities, including infant care for up to forty-eight hours.[44] An epidural may lower your blood pressure, requiring more medical intervention, and it is known to slow down or stall contractions, usually requiring additional medical intervention (Pitocin). Pitocin can cause longer, stronger contractions; it may lead to fetal distress, which may lead to Cesarean birth.

Also, an epidural may cause extreme itching, requiring additional medical intervention which, in turn, may cause nausea and dizziness. It can increase maternal temperature, especially when given early in labor, requiring additional medical intervention for the baby after birth. This may result in the baby being away from the mother for a long period of time. It also may cause or increase nausea, vomiting, and shivering.

It will take away your natural ability to produce endorphins, which are your body's way of naturally coping with labor pressure.

It may strip you of the self-confidence that you will feel if you birth naturally and painlessly using your innate ability. I have seen women unable to recall the birth and the first time they held their baby as a result of an epidural or heavier drug such as the commonly used narcotics (morphine, Demerol, Nubain, or Stadol). These narcotics have a systemic effect throughout the body, which may sedate the newborn child long after she is born. The infant's sedation may affect his rate of breathing and a drug, such as Narcan, may be given to the infant to reverse the effects of the narcotics. You may have to wake up your baby often to feed since he might sleep as a result of the drugs used during labor.

Finally, if an epidural is inserted poorly, you may still feel everything, yet remain confined to the bed and unable to use any other natural coping mechanisms.

The effect of epidural anesthesia on breastfeeding is highly controversial. These difficulties include inability to find the nipple, inability to self-latch, and inability to suck properly. Difficulties in suckling occur because anesthetics enter the mother's circulation and cross the placenta. The newborn's liver is too immature to break down the medication, so the effects linger. "A thorough review of the effect of epidurals and narcotics on subsequent breastfeeding found that epidural drugs are present in the laboring mother's bloodstream, cross the placenta to the fetus and affect the baby's later behavior, often causing difficulty with latching on and "inefficient" sucking. These "sleepy" babies may need more time to "acquire efficient breastfeeding skills."[45]

After an epidural birth, you may experience effects similar to a hangover. You may not be able to attend to your baby's needs the same way you'd be able to if you had been sober.

Consciousness of Consequences

I once had a client who simply didn't want to hear anything negative about pregnancy and birth.[46] I respected her desires, but I was curious as to what her reasoning was for not wanting to know her options. One thing I noticed was that this particular client didn't want to use the training CDs she had received as part of her doula package. She didn't want to meditate at all, and she lamented that the five minutes a day I suggested she dedicate to talking to her baby was something she could never remember to do. She felt strongly about having a natural childbirth and told me she had an aversion to using any drugs. Every time I went to see her during our prenatal visits, I had this funny image of being in front of a little girl who would place her fingers in her ears, chanting "lalalala" as I talked.

First, I thought I was the problem, but then I chose to be detached, allowing her to stay as uninformed as she wanted to be. I made sure to let go of my belief that she needed to know what I wanted her to know. When we got together to do a hypnotherapy session, she had a hard time talking to her baby. She couldn't hear his voice and was actually afraid to listen to any message he might have had. After her due date had come and gone, I suggested she visit an acupuncturist to stimulate labor, but she decided against it.

Unfortunately, her labor never started. The doctor, two weeks after her due date, finally proposed an induction using Pitocin, but her baby didn't respond well to that drug. As soon as the first little contraction came, the baby's heart rate plummeted. Once the Pitocin was turned off, and the mother relaxed, his heartbeat came back to a normal state. It seemed like both the mother and child were just not ready to go through the natural birthing experience. Finally, after attempting Pitocin one more time and witnessing the baby in distress again, her doctor decided that a Cesarean birth was the only way this baby was going to be born. My client's worst nightmare had come true. She had refused to be prepared in case of a Cesarean birth and was now faced with it.

At her bedside, we talked about listening to the baby's clear message: he simply did not like to be forced out. The mother was devastated. She began feeling responsible for the outcome and suddenly she distrusted her doctor. She was filled with questions: Was the doctor making the decision because she wanted to go home? Had she done something wrong? Should she have waited this long before inducing? What other natural way could we use to induce the labor? At this point, it was too late. We talked about accepting what was happening as her child's will. For even a Cesarean birth can be painless as long as there is consciousness and preparation.

After the delivery, the doctor couldn't really tell why the baby had experienced distress. When I came over for my postpartum visit, the mother was once again focusing on why it had not worked out. She was in a frenzy, questioning the doctor's competence and her own actions. We worked on accepting the fact that there are two people responsible for the outcome of a birthing experience and that this time she had to accept that her child had simply opted for his way, not hers. She realized that her fear of a Cesarean had made her totally unconscious during her preparation leading up to the birth. She also realized that regardless of her desires, she needed to respect and accept the desires and choices the baby made. This amazing lesson was life-changing for her. She began working on herself and in her last e-mail she said, "Motherhood comes with a lot of self-actualization and realization. Next time I'll have a VBAC (vaginal birth after Cesarean)."

Sometimes babies decide to come into this world in a different way than we have planned. We must accept and hear their needs and desires and make peace with the fact that all is perfect the way it is. In life, there are no mistakes, only lessons to be learned. If for any reason you end up with a Cesarean birth, don't feel guilty or unfortunate, and don't think there's something wrong with you. Sometimes events in our lives are simply catalysts for our higher good. Success stories are often tales of triumph over trials, and victories over victimizations. Make the experience something you can learn from. Get informed and prepare ahead of time. Your doula or childbirth educator can enlighten you on the most common reasons why a doctor would suggest a Cesarean. Visit www.ican-online.org (International Cesarean Awareness Network) and stay informed. Also visit www.vbac.com to find out about vaginal births after a Cesarean. No matter what the outcome, you can be proud of your birthing experience. My good friend Kathrin, who's also a doula, explains it so well in the following story.

Kathrin's Birth Story

I had a homebirth planned. When my midwife checked me for the first time, I was dilated eight centimeters and we realized the baby was a footling breech (which meant that we had to transfer to the hospital quickly and I was to have a surgical birth). I mourned a lot during the whole process, but somehow overcame my grief. One of the most empowering things I learned was the realization that I still gave birth to my son. In the English language (I'm from Switzerland), people would ask, "Who delivered your baby?" "I did!" was my answer. Other people assisted, but I did give birth. I "delivered" him, I birthed him, and no one else did!

Once I spoke those words out loud, I felt so much better! I felt the power had been given back to me, the power that I felt had been taken away before. When someone asks me the same question now, "Who delivered your baby?" I still speak these words: "I did." I wish we all could be more aware of how we ask women about their births, and that we could let every woman know, no matter how she gave birth, that she was the one giving birth, delivering the baby!

My son is fifteen months old now (so everything is still very fresh in my mind), and I'm ready to have a home-birth with my second child in five weeks!!! Yeah . . . baby!!!

CONSCIOUSNESS AND BREECH BABIES

When treating a breech pregnancy in my hypnotherapy practice, the mom-to-be sometimes exhibits low self-esteem, fear of pain, fear of failure, the need to please others more than herself, and interestingly enough, fear of success. However, one day I discovered yet another fear.

Beth's Story

After repeated insistence from one of her friends, Beth decided to come to me for a hypnotherapy session to see if we could turn her breech baby. As the interview began, I saw that Beth had come more to appease her friend than truly wanting to change the position of her baby. She mentioned that she had tried chiropractic care, but had given up after one visit. She had also turned down her doctor's suggestion for a version at thirty-eight weeks to attempt to turn the baby around. Hypnosis always sheds light on the unknown, but as in this case, the results were very different than expected.

While in a deep state of relaxation, Beth began recounting her own birthing experience. She had been born in the Middle East and due to a complicated set of circumstances, her mother's family left her during labor in the care of a group of women. Beth's mom had tried to concentrate on managing her labor, but the women who surrounded her were accustomed to screaming and chanting in a language that was strange to the laboring woman. Beth remembered the terror she felt as a baby, coming into a room that echoed with a language she did not understand, and feeling her mother's loneliness and fear. Her mother belonged to a tribe that had a tremendous history of violence with the tribe of the women who surrounded her, and hearing the voice of the "enemy" could have also brought up some ancestral terror. This fear from her own birth could have been enough to make her baby go into a breech position. Yet, that didn't seem to be the cause, so we continued searching.

When Beth tried to ask her baby what she felt about turning into a head-down position and being born vaginally, she got no response. At that point, Beth felt compelled to tell me a secret. She explained how a member of her family was very sick and in the hospital. His condition had begun to worsen at almost the same rate as her baby was growing in her womb. He needed a transplant, and another member of the family had volunteered. The entire family had come together to help with the situation and Beth didn't know if any of them would actually be at her birth, because the double operation was going to happen around the time of her due date. Beth suddenly stated, "I can offer this Cesarean to God in exchange for my relative's well-being." She figured that there was a limit to the number of miracles God would allow in her family and that her relative's life was more important than having her desired natural childbirth. The mold was cast, the decision made, and nothing and no one could change it.

When I brought her out of hypnosis, she was relieved and a little surprised. Even though I told her that God has infinite miracles to bestow among his children, I had to accept her decision and supported her newfound peace. Now that she knew why she didn't want her baby to turn around, she felt serene and somehow useful in her family's situation. By sacrificing her right to have a natural childbirth, she firmly believed that she was contributing to the support of the family and her relative's much needed miracle. Just by admitting to herself, to God, and to another human being the exact nature of her decision, she felt better, and this gave her the strength to tell her friend that her having a Cesarean birth was not going to be the end of the world and was part of a bigger plan.

When she left my office, she seemed to be a different person. Her demeanor had changed and she held her head high. The freedom to be vulnerable by confessing what she herself knew was not logical, but was nevertheless her firm decision, had somehow lifted a weight off her shoulders. I heard later that she had given birth to a wonderful baby and was having the time of her life and her relative had survived the transplant. Sometimes we simply need to understand our decisions and have the courage to stand by them.

CONSCIOUSLY VULNERABLE

Living a conscious life means living in the eternal here and now. Existing in the here and now means letting go of any expectations you have for your future, and any memory you have of the past. It means viewing each experience as if it was your first. But most importantly it means allowing yourself to be absolutely vulnerable. When we hear the word *vulnerable,* we immediately think of weakness. Being *vulnerable* is usually associated with opening yourself up to being hurt emotionally and/or physically. But the vulnerability I am talking about is one that requires great courage and strength.

During pregnancy, you've probably been feeling more vulnerable than you've ever felt in your entire life. Being so close to the creator Herself, you're instinctively going toward the highest spiritual manifestation of yourself, which is one of vulnerability. We know that in love, the more open and vulnerable we allow ourselves to be, the more we reach greater depths of intimacy. Becoming a mother is a lifelong love affair. We are most vulnerable when we request, encourage, and welcome honest feedback about ourselves in our quest to live a conscious life, even if such feedback is negative. If you want to experience a painless childbirth, you must be willing to take chances and try new methods, challenges, or behaviors, even though the outcome is unsure. Uncertainty and vulnerability are two characteristics we have fought hard to reject in the modern world.

In the last two hundred years, more and more women have entered the work force and had to take on the warrior archetype. As warriors we constantly battle and compete. In the business world, expressing one's emotion is considered unprofessional and it is looked down upon as a sign of weakness. Women had to learn a new game; they don't show their feelings, they shut down and choose silence over expression, or opt for aggression and defiance. It feels safer to build a wall around us so that no one can come close and hurt us, or dismiss us as weak and unpredictable. We must look detached, in control, rational, and poised. Vulnerability became a fault and women have to assume a role that goes against their very nature. This has been the price women had to pay to become powerful, independent, self-reliant, and successful. Unable to leave work at work, we bring these survival mechanisms home. As women, we are born to multitask. Thus, we have come to believe that we're the only ones who can get things done, and get them done fast enough and perfectly enough. Some of us believe that men cannot handle taking care of a job, a marriage, a house, and kids all at the same time, so we take on the role of superwoman and juggle it all to make it happen. As a result, we often become bitter, angry, and condescending with these inferior males who seem to want it all, yet are incapable of managing any of it, even if we let them. We believe that there's no time to experiment by letting our men take care of the business of holding a family together, and so we regretfully volunteer to do it all ourselves. We can be controlling even when we constantly please or placate others, for we fear that if we let them see our negative side, they won't like what they see. We are frequently on the offensive—attacking, blaming, or correcting others. This keeps the spotlight on others and off ourselves.

When we become mothers and get in touch with the creator within us, we must try new behaviors, attitudes, or beliefs in the pursuit of self-knowledge. In other words, we must let go of the warrior archetype and embrace the mother one and surrender to vulnerability. Tuning into our feelings and learning to express them enables us to have a healthy perspective on ourselves, our problems, and our place in life.

When you become a mother you have become one with the goddess and this new path takes great strength of character and courage. A goddess is the embodiment of the Divine in a female body. She acts with integrity while loving and nurturing. She lets go of anger, pain, fear, guilt, and judgment. She has no need to change anybody and she does not blame, for she sees the Divine in all beings. She has learned to love unconditionally, and has no expectations. She encourages and allows things to be what they are and welcomes other people's efforts, as she looks at everyone the way a mother looks at her child. She knows that life is a mystery that cannot be conquered or understood. She finds her sense of humor, especially about herself, as she feels compassion for all her little idiosyncrasies and human characteristics. She searches for and embraces her Divinity, knowing that change is inevitable and that happiness is found in the journey, not in the end result. Sure this is a tall order, but it is what we strive to become. One day at a time.

As we learn the tools needed to reach a higher state of consciousness we teach and share them first with our child and then with the entire human race. Mastering this journey will make you a living example. Becoming vulnerable will open you up to the heavens. A pebble, big or small, thrown into the water, will ripple a thousand wrinkles in the eternal space and time continuum. Its energy will reach every shore. Your experience shared with other women will be like the pebble reaching women all over the world, strengthening their resolve for a painless and drug-free birth.

Conscious Living

My philosophy teacher one day raised a glass of water and asked us, "How heavy do you think this glass of water is?" The students' answers ranged from six to ten ounces. "Actually, its weight does not depend on how much water there is inside the glass. It depends on how long you hold it. If I hold it for a minute, it is OK. If I hold it for an hour, my right arm will ache. If I hold it for a day, you will have to call an ambulance. It is the exact same weight, but the longer I hold it, the heavier it becomes." She said, "If we carry our burdens all the time, sooner or later, we will not be able to carry on as the burden becomes increasingly heavier. What you have to do is to put the glass down and rest for a while before holding it up again." Whatever burdens you have now on your shoulders, let them down for a moment. You can pick them up again later when you have rested. Or maybe when you feel ready to pick them up again, you'll realize that you no longer have to or want to. Feel how good it is to be free from the burdens you have been carrying, and then notice how the power to be free from them was yours all along.

8

the right to divine powers

As I embrace my relationship with the Divine, abundance and power follow. I relax in the arms of Infinite Love, finding serenity and confidence in its support. Through the power of prayer, meditation, self-hypnosis, and visualization, I am in touch with my Divine and primordial ability to give birth to my child naturally and painlessly. I recognize and affirm my child's Divine nature and I savor the sacredness of the birth that is to come. I give life to another expression of God. By embracing my role as the creator, I consciously participate in bringing the miracle into life. I am grateful and humbled by my right to access what is already mine. I release it into the Spirit; it is done. And so it is. Amen.

YOUR BABY NOW

Your baby is gaining about half a pound per week, and layers of fat are piling on. She has probably turned head-down in preparation for birth. Her brain continues to develop and we could speculate that the baby's brain is now fully functioning and is becoming even more aware of her surroundings. Her lungs are getting close to full maturity and if born now she has a good chance to do well. She can make the distinction between sweet and sour tastes in the amniotic fluid. There is little room in the womb, so movement will be less vigorous, but you can expect her to move frequently.

YOUR BODY

You may tire easily as you go down this final stretch. Some women have trouble sleeping at night; I tell my clients it is Mother Nature's way to prepare you for the sleepless nights ahead. At the end of this month, you will get a Group B Strep test. GBS infections can be successfully treated with antibiotics such as penicillin or ampicillin, given intravenously during labor. You should be feeling Braxton Hicks[47] contractions pretty regularly now. These are a sort of practice contractions. Your uterus is gearing up and exercising for the upcoming event. They are not a cause for concern. Your baby may have dropped down into the pelvis, called lightening or engagement, in preparation for birth. This causes your pelvis to expand, which may cause some pelvic pressure and result in your needing to urinate more often. The ever-increasing size of your baby may also be pushing him up into your rib cage, which may be feeling sore. Consider visiting a chiropractor or a massage therapist to alleviate some of the discomfort.

THE EIGHTH CHAKRA

We have seen how the seven chakras—and the basic human rights ruling them—and the physical development of the fetus have a common denominator. Now in the eighth month of gestation the baby's ability to dream is directly correlated with the eighth chakra and the eighth basic human right to divine power.

In this stage of development, the baby begins experiencing sleep cycles during which rapid eye movement has been observed. David B. Chamberlain, Ph.D., writes, "Researchers have discovered that babies are dreaming when rapid eye movement sleep is first observed." Chamberlain also explains, "Dreaming is a vigorous activity involving apparently coherent movements of the face and extremities in synchrony with the dream itself, manifested in markedly pleasant or unpleasant expressions. Dreaming is also an endogenous activity, neither reactive nor evoked, expressing inner mental or emotional conditions."[48]

Throughout history, dreams have been seen as a type of Divination and a direct connection with God. Stories about dreams and actions that resulted from dreams (sometimes referred to as visions) can be found in most of the world's religious traditions.

In ancient Judeo-Christianity, Jacob, Joseph, and Daniel are given the ability to interpret dreams by Yahweh. In the New Testament, Divine inspiration comes to Saint Joseph, Mary's husband, when the Angel Gabriel tells him in a dream that the baby Mary is carrying is the Son of God. We find sophisticated discussions of dream interpretation in the Talmud, the importance expressed in this quote: "A dream which is not interpreted is like a letter which is not read." Intricate measures for diagnosing and curing illnesses (both physical and psychological) were practiced by tribal shamans among the Diegueno, a Native American people from what is now Southern California.[49] Serenity Young, in her book *Dreaming in the Lotus: Buddhist Dream Narrative, Imagery, and Practice,* tells us that dreams play an essential role in the genre of sacred biography in Indo-Tibetan Buddhism. Dreams are vivid, vital, and meaningful; although we cannot speculate on the nature of our baby's dreams, we know through our own experience that dreams provide highly metaphysical energies. Dreams often speak to our most troubling, conflict-filled concerns, and they offer us guidance, inspiration, and hope. God is communicating directly with our child and our baby's Divine powers are revealed through his ability to dream.

DIVINE POWER OF DREAMS

When we pay attention to the messages of our dreams, we can open a window into our unconscious mind and identify the lessons we need to learn and the fears we need to remove before we birth our baby. One morning, following yet another disturbing dream, I wrote: *non ti vergognare sei meravigliosa!* (Don't feel shamed. You are marvelous!) For years, I had what I used to call nightmares. When everything was going well on the outside, I'd go to sleep and a very painful dream would assail me. My dreams were often staged at an old job where a boss was trying to shame me in some embarrassing moment in front of a lot of people. I used to wake up nearly in tears. The feeling or state I experienced in the dream stayed with me for a whole day. To heal and learn what my unconscious mind was begging me to realize, I began to keep a dream journal. I concentrated on the feelings I experienced, not the images of the dream. I zeroed in on the strong feeling I felt—shame—and using the Feeling Inventory Exercise I found out where the shame had originated from. While growing up phrases evoking shame were often repeated to me not only by my primary caretakers but by the nuns I spent eleven years with. "You should be ashamed of yourself!" was their favorite reprimand. Determined to heal my dreams, I called a hypnotherapist friend and revisited a very important chapter of my life in the nun's convent.

I Want to Be the Madonna

In first grade, the holiday play was traditionally the Nativity. It marked the official rite of passage from babyhood to student. The most sought-out role was the Madonna, followed by the role of the singing, winged angels, whose halos glowed against the starry backdrop. In an all girls school, no one wanted to dress like a boy to play Joseph or one of the magi. Even baby Jesus, though the hero, was still a baby, thus not an appealing part. Lastly, being a shepherd was ridiculed by the children as being the part of a "terrone,"[50] a typical part given to Southerners.

The audition began in the fourth week of school. In preparation, I spent hours in front of the mirror, conjuring up the perfect angelic expression I imagined belonged to the mother of Jesus: eyes positioned low and humble; body posture slightly proud, yet respectful; hands conjoined; azure veil, borrowed from my mom's drawer, pinned below the chin, with head tilted to the left; my shoulders gently turned downward in supplication; and feet together, toes pointed.

Lined up backstage with my classmates, I waited for my turn. I had rehearsed my entrance and walked with grace and deliberation. I took my place next to Joseph and spoke my first line, "Benvenuti." My first grade teacher, Suor Maria Blandina, was distracted by some papers and did not notice me right away. As soon as she heard my voice, she jolted in her seat and barked, "Tornetta, what are you doing there? Do you think Mother Mary would have a nasal voice like yours? How dare you, you should be ashamed of yourself!" I tried to say something, but nothing came out.

"Don't waste my time; you can't possibly think you could be the Madonna. Go, get offstage, and we'll figure out what you can do later." She smiled to her accomplice, the nun at the piano. "Maybe you'll make a good shepherd." My throat closed down, the air trapped, my legs paralyzed. All I could do was stare into her eyes, lips parted, chin quivering. Her words had penetrated my chest, holding and squeezing my heart. I could hear the faint, faraway sound of my classmates laughing at me. Finally, an assistant nun approached and escorted me off stage. The seed of shame followed by pure hatred sprouted in my six-year-old heart.

I ran offstage, into the corridors in the direction of the closest bathroom, while a few girls ran after me singing that litany, "Giuditta parla col naso."[51] Suor Maria Blandina had given a powerful weapon to my classmates, something they used to make fun of me for the next five years. I locked myself in the stall and jumped on the toilet seat. I resolved never to come out of that bathroom. Never! I shouldn't cry, I wouldn't cry, I couldn't allow myself to cry. Suddenly the bell rang—I was saved. All I had to do was grab my coat and run as fast as my feet could carry me to the fence at the bottom of the driveway, where I prayed my mom would not be late.

God answered my prayers. Mom was punctual. I climbed into her car and fearing being punished for having dishonored my family, I tried to pretend everything was fine. "Nini? Cosa c'è?"[52] Feeling safe finally, I began to sob and told my mom what had happened at the audition. With every word, she became more and more enraged.

The family honor was in jeopardy, and something needed to be done. "Don't worry, your father will take care of everything," she resolved. Terror smacked me across the face. Dad, the growling mastiff, would be unleashed.

Wanting to hide, I asked my mom if I could take a nap, and walked to my room longing for my pillow and blanket. At eight o'clock, the front door opened. Dad was home. I closed my eyes tightly, wishing I could vanish. I sensed the rage overtaking the entire house, a dark cloud obscuring the sun, chills running down my back as the air became colder and darkness enveloped all.

"Where is she?" my father roared, running to my bedroom after he was told what had happened at school. Flinging the door open, he shouted, "Tell me everything!" From the corner of my bed, holding tightly to my pillow, I began telling him what had happened. He demanded I go through the details, over and over again: what I had done specifically, what the nun said precisely, and what I had said.

"It is very important for a Tornetta to know how to act in similar situations!" he exclaimed. "The best defense in life is attack, my little one. If you attack the enemy first, the element of surprise will give you the upper hand." I couldn't really understand what he was talking about, but he had finally calmed down and was now sitting on my bed. I inched closer to see if I could steal a hug from him. I really wanted one!

I asked him to tell me a story to show me what he meant. He told me that once a large man had approached him in the street shouting. Without thinking twice, my dad, who was quite a short man, laid the fellow flat on his back with one single butt of his head, putting an immediate stop to the insults. I sneaked into his lap and a second seed was planted: revenge. Sweet, cuddling revenge, just like his arms. I had just found my executioner.

The day after, I was kept home. Dad went to my

school to straighten things out. School friends told me that my dad waited until school let out to attack the nun verbally in front of all the other teachers and the parents who were coming to pick up their children. He ranted and raved and swore and insulted her, the school, and her God. It took a long time to calm him down. When I went to school the following day, kids pointed at me and talked amongst themselves, as did many of the nuns. The whispers grew louder and louder in my head. Everyone knew I was the daughter of that lunatic who had come and used the name of God in vain. I was the daughter of the one who had insulted a little, defenseless nun in the middle of the afternoon. None knew or cared to find out why my dad had been so enraged. Children began making fun of my nasal voice and my first nickname was coined: Nasal Judy.

As the holidays approached, my part in the play had to be decided. The nuns were concerned; certainly, I would not be a shepherd, for they didn't want to suffer another visit from the madman. I couldn't be an angel; after all, angels dwell in heaven and I clearly came from hell. The decision was made by Suor Maria Blandina that a new character was to be present at the Nativity: Mary Magdalene. She mentioned that she had become one of the most important female figures in Jesus' life. She read in class how Mary Magdalene had been the first to see Jesus reincarnate. I was elated! Only later did I learn I had been cast as the whore.

The shame I experienced as a child entrenched itself deeply in my subconscious. Those recurring nightmares were simply a Divine way to communicate to me the need to work on releasing the belief that God was a punishing and shaming force that would penalize me for my thoughts. Thus, if a negative thought would pass through my mind, I was told to be ashamed of myself, for the mere act of imagining something sinful made me a sinner. As a child, I can't tell you how many negative, vindictive thoughts I conjured up, all accompanied by feelings of shame and a constant fear of Divine punishment. This silly and painful conundrum had been abandoned by my adult-self many years ago, but to my surprise, it lingered in my subconscious and would manifest itself through my dreams. Once I found out that this last effigy of my childhood was creeping into my dreams, I had no idea how I could rid myself of it. I had plenty of tools for behavior modification in my wakeful and conscious state, but I felt helpless when it came to dreams I had absolutely no control over.

If I believed that the Mother was communicating with me through my dreams, then I could embrace my Divine right to surrender my shame to Her, and ask Her to remove it.

FORGIVENESS IS THE ANSWER

How was I going to forgive the nun that hurt me so deeply? After all, I could forgive my parents by diving into the love I felt for them, but there was not much love when it came to those who had emotionally scarred me. Once again, I had to appeal to my innate Divine powers, for if God can forgive anyone, I had to find a way to do the same.

I had no idea why this particular nun had been so harsh on me, and so I went back to that audition with my adult-self. I sat down near that nun, realizing I needed to be careful not to insult her or take revenge on her, for that would not have yielded the kind of healing I was after. So, I just put my arms around her and told her that she might not realize it, but what she was about to do to little Giuditta would scar her for years to come. In my vision, she looked at me in puzzlement and said, "I didn't know." Indeed, she must not have really thought of the dire consequences of her actions. She herself must have had such a hurt soul to behave that way with little children. I saw her under a new light and realized that having little, challenging Giuditta in her class must not have been that easy. Maybe I reminded her of someone who had injured her, or maybe she envied my free spirit. Whatever the reason, I was able to look into this nun's eyes and see her pain. I simply let go of the years of shame I felt as a result of that first incident that marked the beginning of a war I fought with her for five long years. I shed many tears for the hurt I had felt and carried for decades, and as I cried, I felt the weight of the old shame lifted. I took responsibility for hanging onto that particular episode and embraced the circumstances that had created such an event. In the end, I was glad I had the experience, for without it, I would not have learned how to forgive using my innate Divine powers.

During pregnancy many women have very vivid dreams. Whether good or challenging, you must pay attention to them. As creators of another human life our sense of intuition is extremely heightened. I had a client who dreamed she was going to have a little girl, even before she conceived, and my son came to me in a dream in the early days of my pregnancy to tell me his name.

When you hear of the prophetic quality of dreams, you may be afraid of what your dreams are prophesying for the future. Have no fear, for dreams are loving teachers that can either reward you with prophecy or get your attention with a nightmare, but they will never punish you. In this time leading up to the birthing event, keep a dream journal on your bedside and jot down the feelings you have experienced throughout the night. If you encounter strong feelings of fear, terror, shame, loss, or rejection, use the Feeling Inventory Exercise and then ask your Higher Power to heal those feelings. Your unconscious is trying to get your attention and, in its desire to heal before the birthing experience, it's sending you a message.

FEAR

The feeling of fear is the most common feeling that comes up in dreams during pregnancy. It's important to recognize the fact that fear that has yet to be dealt with can affect the quality and length of your labor and delivery.[53] Scientific studies indicate that certain hormonal changes take place in the presence of fear, stress, and anxiety. "The adrenaline released while in fear or stress has been referred to as the antithesis of oxytocin, the naturally produced hormone that stimulates uterine contractions. Another category of hormones called catecholamines (which include epinephrine, norepinephrine, and dopamine) is indicated by other studies as one of the causative factors in fetal distress and problematic labor. Catecholamines circulate when the pregnant mother is anxious or afraid, and they pass through the placenta to the baby, affecting his environment."[54]

We know that we tend go into an automatic fight-or-flight reaction in which we tense every muscle of our body in order to prepare for a defensive action. Consequently, fear can be a deciding factor affecting our overall experiences.

- In labor: fear creates tension and tension creates pain.
- In postpartum: fear creates confusion, anxiety, and the feelings of helplessness and of being lost and alone.
- In life: fear is the very obstacle to our self-confidence and, ultimately, to our success.

Be grateful: your dreams help you discover hidden fears and give you a chance to face them. Babies can and will accrue memories while in the womb and will feel and

WE NEED TO ALWAYS REMEMBER THAT MOTHERS WHO ARE AFRAID TEND TO SECRETE THE HORMONES THAT DELAY OR INHIBIT BIRTH. THIS IS TRUE OF ALL MAMMALS AND IS PART OF NATURE'S DESIGN. THOSE WHO ARE NOT TERRIFIED ARE MORE LIKELY TO SECRETE IN ABUNDANCE THE HORMONES THAT MAKE LABOR AND BIRTH EASIER AND LESS PAINFUL—SOMETIMES EVEN PLEASURABLE.

INA MAY GASKIN,
INA MAY'S GUIDE TO CHILDBIRTH

embrace the mother and father's emotions. If fear and low self-esteem are what you feel most of the time, so will your child.

Learn to embrace your fears, because trying to erase them will only make them fight harder to survive.

Imagine a small child, frightened and shaky, screaming under the covers at the monster she believes lives in the closet. Mom runs into the room, "What's the matter? Don't be silly! There are no monsters in the closet." This answer won't appease the child. In fact, being dismissed and ridiculed will cause the fear to hide deep within the child's unconscious. The child resolves to not share her fears with Mom to avoid being belittled and ridiculed. Ideally the scene could go as follows:

Mom walks in and hugs the child, saying, "So, my little one, tell me more about the monster in the closet." The little girl might respond, "It's big and scary! Make him go away, Mommy!" Then Mom responds by taking her daughter's words seriously, "Do you want me to go and look in the closet and tell him to leave you alone?" "Can you do that?" says the little girl, still frightened. "Sure. In fact, I'm going to leave my angel with you, and together with your angel they'll watch over you." Then Mom shines a light into the closet and speaks these words: "I know you are there, monster, and I want you to know that you are frightening my girl. From now on, my angel and her angel will stand guard over her so you may not come back here and frighten her."

Simply denying ours or our children's fears and negative feelings will only make them stronger. Through the lesson learned in the second chakra associated with our right to feel, we have learned that we need to acknowledge our feelings, even those that seem unjustified or fantastic, like the fear of the monster in the room.

In this book, we are learning to parent ourselves so that we may learn how to parent our child. Using our dreams as a tool for knowledge will bring us closer to the realization that we have within us Divine powers to heal ourselves and others, and to love unconditionally all that was, is, and will be.

WHO AND WHAT IS MY GOD

Before we can find the right to Divine power within us we need to define what our Higher Power, or a power greater than ourselves is. Do you have a clear concept of your Higher Power, or have you been borrowing images and concepts conjured up by others?

How do you apply the principles of this book if you can't feel a connection with the Divine? If you consider yourself an agnostic (a person who can neither deny nor confirm the existence of God) or have doubts, I suggest you consider turning your will and your life over to the natural flow of things, the laws of nature, and unconditional love. If you agree that your life could use some conscious and deliberate living, and you agree that you cannot do all this by yourself, then you agree that you need help from a more powerful source then yourself. You don't need to worship a particular God, or associate with any particular religion. The very act of letting go of resentments, self-pity, fear, and whatever else keeps your thoughts going in circles, is a spiritual solution without denomination, one that will empower you with the laws of nature. When we appeal to God in our affirmations, we simply ask ourselves to be a good person, a better person, to remove from us a character defect placed there unconsciously at one point or another in our lives. What is a "good person?" One who focuses on doing the very best she can, staying honest with herself and others, and committing to heal and parent herself. As we live this way we teach our children the tools that will lead them to their own divine powers.

As you have gained self-confidence in your own ability to bring forth this baby painlessly and naturally, you are now a vessel for the Divine power of creation to operate through.

I invite you to list the qualities of your Higher Power in order to get closer to your personal connection and recognize some of the ways you experience the divine. Some of our beliefs about God no longer serve us in our intention to have a painless childbirth and to live consciously. Some of us have been taught of a God that can be punishing and fickle. One who rewards only those who have done well. Then there is an unpredictable and unreliable one, who has limited power, who is absent when you need Him, and who only takes care of His favorites. If God is ideal and He is perfect then these anthropomorphic qualities are not His. God resonates as the Divine qualities of unconditional love and gratitude, not fear and revenge.

DIVINE CREATIVE PROCESS

An ideal is the concept of something in its state of absolute excellence and perfection. No matter what our nationality, religion, or spiritual philosophy is we have some universal agreements of ideals. For example, it's safe to say that we all agree it would be ideal if there was more love, peace, beauty, and joy in the world. Similarly, it's safe to assume that all women would agree that a painless childbirth is the ideal way to bring a baby into this world. When we consider ideals we often look at them as utopic, impossible, and even child-ish dreams. Of course, we'd like to see peace on earth, but will it ever really happen? To say, "People will always fight and there will always be wars," is looking at the glass half empty. On the other hand, to say, "Love, peace, and joy on earth start at home," is a step toward changing the world. Tackling the big problems by taking a series of small steps makes the ideal seem possible. The secret to having a pain-less childbirth is no different: one change at a time, one con-traction at a time. Being a woman and a mother, you have an amazing, innate gift: intuition. We need to let go of our rational mind, which can often be judgmental and cynical, if we want to manifest our ideal. In the English dictionary, intuition is defined as: direct perception of truth, fact, inde-pendent of any reasoning, yet dependent on *faith*. Intuition is not a left brain activity; in fact, it often exists in our hearts and in our trust in the Divine. We intuitively know that God is good and that if God is good, it is Her good pleasure to see that Her daughter (you) experiences a painless childbirth. Several anthropologists who have studied primitive tribes around the world have reported that, for the most part, they have witnessed birth not only as a quick and natural event, but as a painless one too.

Joseph Chilton Pearce, in his book *Evolution's End*, writes about Ugandan women giving birth, "The optimum length for birthing seems to be about twenty minutes." When such a phenomenon is observed, scientists take a look at the envi-ronment surrounding the pregnant woman, the beliefs of the entire tribe, and her expectations. The cultural beliefs mirror the outcome. Thanks to our culture, we have been taught the opposite, and so it is important that we use a leap of faith in a loving Mother Nature to obtain our ideal—a painless childbirth.

From this faith an idea emerges: I am going to have a painless childbirth. Begin to visualize the birthing experience in all its details and hold these images in your mind. See who, what, where, and with whom you want to experience this birth. Create vivid images, and bring them into your daily meditation practice. Soon, as you become accustomed to these constant visions of a painless childbirth, you experience feelings of accomplishment, as if the ideal birth has already happened. This practice is used widely by athletes. Before the race, they continuously envision the event in detail and imagine not only participating in it, but winning. They go into the feeling of ripping apart the ribbon at the finishing line as they hear the audience roar in excitement.

The more you experience your dream, the more your psyche believes it has already happened. Nothing will stand in the way of your confidence. By staying inspired (in-spirit) during these visualizations, you are moved to action. All the actions you take during your pregnancy become a result of the process you are going through, from ideal to imagination, from inspiration to action. The actions can be random or calculated. Reading this book is an action. Having conversations with other women who have had a similar experience, or accidentally meeting someone who stirs you in the direction of a doctor, midwife, or hypnotherapist, are also actions. From this high sense of conscious creation of your lives, all meetings and all communications are no longer random; you are attracting into your life that which you need and/or desire. In essence, you have become an irresistible magnet for all that belongs to you, claiming your right to your Divine powers.

Finally the big day is upon you, you are in labor, and as you have lived for nine months in an inspired, in-spirit state, you experience the birthing you have visualized. I had a client who had imagined going on a walk at the beach with her husband to view the sunset while in labor. She called me from the beach and told me she was in labor and was watching the sunset. Her birth visualization was unfolding exactly as she had dreamed it would.

One would think that the manifestation of a painless childbirth would be the end of the creative process; actually, it is the beginning of the new life, the mother and child's. Once we have experienced the manifestation of our desires, we are conscious of our reactions. Depending on the birthing experience you've gone through, unless you become conscious of your life and actions, you will have an equal experience with your child and your life after the birth.

The feelings that come about after you give birth to your baby are very important. Mothers who have had a natural childbirth often feel a greater sense of accomplishment and seldom fall into depression. After birthing their baby, they tend to feel uplifted and joyful. Yes, it is true that their hormones will be raging, and that at times tears will stream down their face for seemingly no reason, but I don't call this the baby blues. This is the opening of the heart.

No matter what your birth was like, begin immediately with the feeling of gratitude. Be grateful that it is over. Be grateful for having a painless birthing experience, or because your baby is so beautiful, or your partner so loving, or your new family so cute and adorable. No matter what, at this point you have gained greater knowledge of the process. This will be an invaluable treasure for your next pregnancy.

Having manifested your heart's desires brings you to the recognition that you indeed can do it. There is a fundamental spiritual law that says if one can do it, we all can. The first woman to run in the Olympics set a record of speed and time. She was surely followed by the next woman who broke that record, and so on. By the time a few years passed, the record had been broken with numbers that would have been unimaginable at the beginning. Once one woman broke the "mold," many more followed. Once you have achieved your desired birthing experience, you have become an instrument of God's power of creation and one with the creative force. This great wisdom and recognition of the absolute Divine ideal must be shared. Become a painless childbirth advocate; share the joy with all you see.

Alexander the Great

Kevin and Ellen are two young, beautiful people who, while pregnant with their first child, lost both their jobs and their home. Ellen called me in labor; they had just become homeless. There was no fear in her voice, no worry. She simply stated she was confident they would be taken care of by the Divine.

None of the shelters we called had room for them, so I let them stay with me on Wednesday night. On Thursday, we woke up and went to Ellen's doctor. Ellen was four centimeters dilated and 80 percent effaced. The doctor said he wanted her at the hospital right away; he would break her waters and induce labor. She had preeclampsia earlier in this pregnancy and had already been at the hospital for two weeks on bed rest. Despite their situation, Kevin and Ellen were beaming. I never once heard Ellen complain or talk about fear of not having a place to stay, and there was no tension or blame between the two of them. They were simply dedicated to the moment at hand, and right now, despite the circumstances, the only task they wanted to concentrate on was the birth of their baby. Alexander the Great, as they called him, was ready to come into the world and both mom and dad knew the Divine would provide.

We decided to take our time before we went to the hospital. We were all hungry, so we went back to my house and had a lovely lunch where we got to know each other a bit better. I showed them a few videos to visually prepare Ellen for the labor, and then we took a walk on the beach. When I encouraged Ellen to tell Kevin how she wanted to be supported during labor, they laughed and cuddled as they prepared for the event.

We drove to the hospital in the afternoon and arrived around 4:00 p.m. The attending nurse was very encouraging, and she quickly became part of our team.

Waters were broken at 5:15 p.m., and shortly thereafter, Ellen's contractions gently grew stronger. She was in good spirits and promised me she would surprise us all and laugh all the way into delivery.

By 7:00 p.m., she was nine centimeters and 100 percent effaced. Ellen walked to the delivery room, slowly dancing in Kevin's arms, managing the contractions. She was still smiling. A short half an hour later, she was ready to hug her baby out. We tried to squat, but the nurse was too worried; she thought that such fast progress would bring the baby so soon, it would birth on the floor. When I suggested we put the mattress on the floor, she looked at me as if I were from outer space. I had gone a bit too far even for a supportive nurse. So we helped Ellen onto the bed, and with Kevin on one side and me on the other, she began breathing her baby out. ALEXANDER THE GREAT graced our planet. Ellen let out a faint laugh just to show me she was still capable of laughing all the way through. Kevin was in tears and in love.

When the baby was placed on Ellen's stomach, her doctor walked in, jokingly reprimanding Ellen for not having waited for her and having delivered the baby with the resident doctor. But upon finding out both new parents were homeless, she offered them her own home. Ellen's

Divine powers were exhibited through her manifestation, not only for a painless childbirth and a place to labor with her husband before she came to the hospital, but by finding the type of provider who would go far beyond anyone's expectations and offer her own house to the new family. A week later, Ellen's mom came in from Michigan to take Ellen and the baby back home until Kevin found a house. No reprimand, no judgment. This family was kept together and safe through their own Divine powers.

OTHER PEOPLE'S DIVINE POWERS

There is a story in the Bible (Mark 2:1–12) about a man who was completely paralyzed. One day, Jesus came to a village nearby and the news of his gift of healing spread rapidly. Four friends offered to carry the paralyzed man to meet Jesus to plead for his help. Some Bible scholars believe that they walked three miles to reach their destination. When they arrived, a great crowd stood outside Jesus' residence. At first glance, it seemed impossible to make their way through all these people. I imagine the man in the stretcher thought that there were other people more deserving than himself among the crowd. But his friends' determination was so strong that, carrying the stretcher on their shoulders, they climbed up onto the roof, looking for an alternate entrance. Once on the roof, they saw a small opening into the house. Determined to give their friend a chance at a miracle, they dug with their bare hands through tiles and dirt to enlarge the hole on the roof.

> You can have anything you want in your life if you help others get what they want.
>
> Zig Zigler

Finally, when the hole was big enough to fit their friend through, they saw Jesus' eyes watching them. They smiled and, as the Bible says, "When Jesus saw their faith," he said to the paralytic " . . . get up, take your mat and go home." The faith and dedication of the paralytic's friends was rewarded.

We have all had difficult times, and we get paralyzed by fear, worry, and depression. In these times, whom do you rely on? Who are the people in your life who would lay down their lives for you, who believe in you, who know you deserve the best, and who would go to bat for you?

Rejoice! Some day soon, your child will be one of those people. She will be someone who will carry you, tearing down obstacles with her bare hands to make sure Mom gets what she needs. She will tell you, "Mom, you'll make it through this, we are going to make it together. Everything is going to be all right."

Astro's Birth, by Justine

Friday, four days before my due date, I had a checkup at my doctor's office. It was around 11:00 a.m., and by the time I left at 1:00 p.m., I was headed home to grab my bags and go straight to the hospital to get induced. My doctor said that my fluid was starting to get low, and that she didn't want to wait over the weekend, in case something happened to the baby. I was absolutely torn. My heart had been set on spending most of my labor at home and only going to the hospital near the end. I trusted that I would go into labor at the right time. At the same time, my doctor was recommending this course of action, and I worried that something could happen to the baby. Right now, he was doing well and I could hear his heartbeat, but what if it stopped? I was afraid.

I cried all the way home. By 5:00 p.m., I was in a hospital bed with my partner Arno at my side, and they started the Pitocin drip. I had talked to our doula, Giuditta, a number of times. I could tell she didn't feel inducing at this stage (four days before the due date, with no real problems) was the best course of action, but I still felt completely supported by her, and that gave me strength.

Around 6:00 p.m., my blood pressure was skyrocketing and they gave me a magnesium drip to prevent seizures. It made me feel hot, sweaty, and nauseated. Because it is a muscle relaxant, they would not let me stand up or get out of bed. It was really frustrating because I had envisioned relaxing in my bathtub at home, and moving and walking in the ways that felt natural to me. I felt like I had stepped into a machine and that I had to fight every step not to get swept up in the conveyor belt where all decisions would be made for me, and I would be spit out the other end, having been processed.

Around 7:00 p.m., Arno commented that we had been there for only three hours and already I had three IVs in one arm and a blood pressure cuff attached to the other. Every new nurse that came in would begin with, "When are you getting your epidural?" or "Are you ready for your epidural?" I had to say "NO, NO, NO," and more "NO's." Beforehand, I had decided I wanted to try to do it without one, but if I couldn't, I would use an epidural and not feel bad about it. As the night progressed, I was having stronger and stronger contractions, but I felt like I was managing well and didn't need one at that point. The fact that they kept bugging me about it and expected me to get one strengthened my resolve.

Arno was so sweet and helped me all night long. We had a routine where he would spray my face with water and give me ice chips. He also helped me with the bedpan so that we wouldn't have to call the nurse. Throughout the night, every so often we would hear a new baby crying and would think, "Where is ours?" By 6:00 a.m., I was feeling I must be getting pretty close. My contractions were very strong; I was guessing that I was about eight centimeters dilated. When they checked me, I was still only one centimeter dilated. This was the hardest time during the delivery. Everyone was talking about a Cesarean, and I was so tired I just didn't care anymore. They took me off the Pitocin to let me rest and get ready for a C-section.

I spoke to Giuditta, who reminded me that I had options. She suggested I tell the nurse that I wanted to speak to my doctor. It was now about 7:00 a.m. The nurse got my doctor on the phone, and she was leaning toward a Cesarean birth. When I asked her if there were any other options, she suggested we try another drug, this time a cervix softener. I was really uncomfortable with adding another drug to the mix, especially one that could not be turned off. I asked her to come in and examine me and then we would together decide what to do. She got there in a few hours and upon examination, she found that I had scar tissue on my cervix that was holding my cervix closed. After she broke up the scar tissue with her fingers, she said she was hopeful that I could have a vaginal delivery. I asked if we could just try the Pitocin again since I was having strong contractions with it. She agreed to try it, but I was first given a four-hour break. I tried to eat a piece of French toast, but it came right back up, and I tried to sleep, but it was impossible.

We were set to try again starting at noon. The doctor thankfully had me moved to a delivery room that was much nicer than the room we had been in. Giuditta was on her way, and things were looking up. When she arrived, she said "Let's just forget about yesterday and start fresh now, as if you've just arrived at the hospital." We put on some Indian music and turned down the lights. I could hear Astro's heartbeat on the monitor; it sounded like a racehorse, fast and steady. From then on, things were much better. Arno and I regained our sense of humor, which meshed very well with Giuditta's. We got a great nurse who had worked with her before. Giuditta talked to me about taking my powers back, managing my own birth and the rate of Pitocin given to me, changing my outlook on how long it had been, and focusing on the job at hand.

I asked the nurse to up the Pitocin slowly so that I could acclimate to the contractions as they increased. She was great, but after her shift ended, I had new nurses who just came in without talking to me and increased the dosage. I had to ask them every time to please respect our wishes. They didn't seem too happy about it.

Finally, I was in active labor. With the use of hypnosis suggestions, I managed to have a pretty good time. I think the hypnosis really relaxed Arno, too. It felt like we were climbing a mountain and Giuditta was our guide or sherpa. It was physically and mentally strenuous, but not painful. During contractions, I had to focus, and in between contractions we relaxed and made jokes. There was not one moment that I felt out of control or like I couldn't do it. There was not one moment I considered an epidural or other pain medication. My fear beforehand was that I would be suffering and really wanting one and going through the agony of trying to not have one. It wasn't like that at all. About a week before, I had watched a hypno-birthing video, and all the moms looked so calm and relaxed. I knew that was how I wanted to be, and so I was. When I looked at the clock, I was shocked that an hour had gone by, then another two hours; it seemed like only fifteen minutes. I tried to stand during some of the contractions to get the help of gravity, though I felt a bit weak because of the magnesium. Arno held me and we did this sort of slow dance movement.

I don't think I realized when I was in transition because I expected it to be more dramatic and more frightening. The contractions were very strong and I vocalized through them. Giuditta showed me how to do a relaxing sound, the sound Ah. I could really feel the difference. Giuditta did more hypnosis at that point and it all went really fast. I started getting some pain in my rear end, so she had me get on all fours with my head lower than my rear end, and this helped the baby back up a bit. Then she put a blanket under my stomach and stood over me, pulling back and forth on the ends. She did this a few times and it wiggled the baby in the right direction.[55] When I sat up, the pain was gone. Now, I just had an incredible urge to push. They checked me and indeed it was time. I did the "no pushing breathing," but I was worried the baby would come before the doctor. I kept talking about the incredible urge I had, and she kept telling me, "Yes, I know, that is what it feels like to have a baby." I couldn't believe it. Finally, the doctor came and it was time. It took me two sets of contractions to realize I didn't know what the hell I was doing. I focused on what Giuditta was saying. They asked me if I wanted a mirror and I said, "No, I'm way too busy for a mirror!" I didn't need one anyway, because I was literally having an out-of-body experience. I could see myself from the ceiling on the other side of the room, from over the doctor's shoulder. When Astro crowned, I was completely aware of it. It stung a little, like a paper cut, and I remember thinking, "Hey, what about the ring of fire?" Arno was so excited, he had a huge smile on his face and was bobbing up and down on his tippy toes. I gave two more pushes and Astro was out at 1:24 a.m. on Sunday morning.

The first thing that Arno said was, "He's so cute," and he was right. Astro was perfect.

Trust

It is not hope I ask from you. Hope conceals the possibility of failure. It is not faith, for that too is too ephemeral, too hard to grab hold of and pocket. I ask yourself to trust with all your might, with your entire body and soul. Trust that you know all there is to know. Trust that the wisdom of the Mother is within you. Trust fully that when the time comes, you will rise to the occasion. Nothing is ever given to us that we cannot handle. God would not have made women go through childbirth without giving us the tools to manage it. Trust that you are a perfect mother, trust that your body will perform to its highest potential, trust that the baby knows her way out. Trust, simply trust, then let go of all control and relax into the ride of your life. When you truly trust, beloved, worries will melt away, tension will be unknown, and the miracle will come forth joyfully and painlessly. Divine Mother will be there with you; just close your eyes and look at Her. You can do this together, you and She. Trust Her, take Her hand, hold on tight, and let go.

the right to be one with the miraculous

The time has come, the tools learned, my child is nearly here. I am one with the Creator; I am filled with integrity and inner wisdom. I stand by my decisions; I call upon my heightened sense of intuition, and I accept that all that will be is exactly as it is supposed to be. I can never be separate from the source. Therefore, I can never be separate from all that God is: infinite wisdom, unconditional love, painless childbirth, balance, abundance, right action, and joy. I am ready to be a vessel of God's life, I am here to give life the Divine incarnate. Thankfully, I let it be. And so it is. Amen.

YOUR BABY NOW

Your baby is a hefty six to eight pounds, and measures between eighteen and twenty-two inches. As she becomes more crowded, you may feel her move around less. Your baby continues to grow and mature, and the lungs are nearly fully developed. Fingernails and toenails are developing and the external ears are formed. The beginnings of teeth are also forming. During this month, your baby gains about half a pound a week and usually drops into a head-down position and rests lower in your abdomen. Your breathing should be easier once the baby drops, but you'll have to urinate more often because of the pressing on your bladder. Swelling of the ankles and feet may increase. Your cervix will open up (dilate) and thin out (efface) as it prepares for birth. You may be very uncomfortable because of the pressure and weight of the baby. Be sure to rest often.

Did you know that if you're having a girl, you're also holding your future grandchildren in your womb? Little girls are born with all their eggs already present in their ovaries, so your future granddaughter or grandson and their life potential is already within you. Isn't that a miraculous legacy?

THE NINTH CHAKRA

The ninth chakra is connected to being one with the divine. This chakra is the other angel hovering over mom's shoulder. It serves as a reminder that the divine will incarnate and come through you at the time of the birth. During your nine months of gestation, as you have done the work suggested in this book, you have added depth to your life. You embody the beauty and attraction of a woman who is ready to follow through with her life's purpose. You have knowledge and you have set your intentions, and now you are ready to embrace and become one with the miraculous.

According to observation,[56] your baby's brain is fully functioning. If born any time past the thirty-sixth week of gestation, he'll have a good chance to thrive. With all physical needs met, he is ready to come into this world and be the creator of his own reality. Last month we saw how, through dreams, he began connecting with the Divine. This month he is becoming his own expression of the most high. Your baby is becoming conscious of himself. All you have to do is surrender to the natural course of things, be the vessel for the miracle to unfold, and your hard work will pay off. You can share with your child what it feels like to be one with the divine.

THE RIGHT TO BE ONE WITH THE DIVINE

Many illustrious men and women spend time in contemplation and come out of it renewed, restored, and prepared to fulfill their destiny. They are born into this world to become immortal teachers. Moses was in contemplation for forty years, Confucius for three, Jesus for forty days, and Mother Teresa prayed for six years before she decided to become a nun.

You had nine months. We have been offered a great destiny to fulfill and it is important. Every woman who embraces the nine months of pregnancy as a conscious contemplation, a period to come closer to the Divinity of creation, a time to learn about herself, her Higher Power, and the world around her, will be ready for the magic unfolding at birth.

What does it mean to be one with the creator? Will I have to give up me to be one with IT? No, you do not lose yourself when you embrace the oneness; instead you gain the Divine. Once you have learned to access and become one with your Higher Power, your only requisite is to name your desire.

The result of that desire is compelled to seek you out. One of the characteristics of Divine power is "all needs are met." Thus, when you feel part of IT, you'll feel part of a universe that rallies for your own good.

God would not have made you capable of bringing into this world a child if the only way to do it was through excruciating pain. Birth is our Divine right; it is the one moment when every woman becomes one with the creator. Focusing on this oneness with God in any occasion will allow the sensation of pain to dissipate because there can't be pain where God is.

As in most traditions, when it comes to explaining the meaning of union with the God, one of the most efficient ways is the use of metaphors. Here is an ancient Hindu tale, coming from the oral tradition, that will give you an inkling of what the union is all about.

A Mother's Tale for Her New Child

"Mommy, where do we come from?"

"That is a good question. Come here honey, sit down, and let me tell you a story . . .

"In the beginning, there was Brahman. Brahman always was, is, and always will be.

"One day, while passing his time alone as usual, he realized that he had so much love inside his heart, he wanted to share it with another. He thought, 'What if I go to sleep and dream of a whole universe, a place where there are skies and seas and trees and animals and flowers.' He began thinking of all the beautiful things he could create in his dream, and that made him very happy.

"Then, he thought, 'If I really want to enjoy this dream and experience all of these wonders that I have created, I must place myself inside this universe.' That, he decided, was a very good idea. 'Yes,' he said, 'I will go to sleep, I will dream of a universe, I will place myself inside it, I will call myself Atman, and I will experience, first-hand, all of the beautiful things I have created. Atman, yes, that is definitely a good name!'

"He smiled to himself and began walking around, feeling out his new name: Atman. Atman. He was quite excited about his idea and broke his walk into a skip of joy, proud of his cleverness. Then, suddenly, he stopped in his tracks, thinking, 'Wait, if I go to sleep and dream of a universe and place myself inside it, as I am, I will know that I created it and I will be unable to savor the illusion.' That disappointed Brahman. The illusion, he thought, wouldn't be an exciting experience; it would just be an illusion.

"He began pacing again and threw himself into deep concentration. 'What if I go to sleep, dream of a universe, place myself inside it, call myself Atman, and take away my memory?' he proposed. The excitement overwhelmed him, and he began jumping up and down, smiling from ear to ear. 'This just might work,' he thought. 'I will not know I am the creator of all things and I will be able to explore and wonder at all the things in the universe.'

"He trembled with excitement and continued to analyze his careful plan, searching for any flaw in it. 'But if I take away my memory, I might never wake up. What if the universe I dream about turns out to be a nightmare?' he asked. That possibility was quite real and quite scary, too. He began pacing again, trying to figure out what to do. 'What to do . . . ? What to do . . . ?'

"'I've got it!' he exclaimed. 'I will go to sleep, I will dream of a universe, I will place myself inside it, I will call myself Atman, I will take away my memory, but I will place clues throughout it to remind myself who I really am, in case I want to wake up.' He was pleased with himself and finally closed his eyes and drifted off to sleep."

"Mama, is he still asleep?"

"Well, my love, Brahman is still asleep, but he does wake up at times. He has had great adventures about which you will hear all your life. Now, let me tell you a secret. I want you to know something. You see . . .

"Your name is Atman. And this is your first clue."

Pregnant with My Daughter

It was Azzurro's first birthday. He was the light of my life, always smiling, always happy. He was walking confidently by then and loved his pasta. Bruce and I had invited some friends over and were celebrating this glorious day. Once everyone had left the party and we put our very tired little boy to sleep in his crib, we went to our bedroom. We retold the story of our son's birth to each other and came together in a loving embrace. It had taken me a little while, but right after falling in love with my son, I had fallen in love with Bruce and we got married. I had longed to be with him so much that that night I'd paid little attention to birth control. I recall feeling the exact moment of conception, our DNA colliding and the new life sprouting inside of me; this time it was pure love. This soul had chosen not to challenge our destiny; she'd come to change my life, show me my purpose, and be a joy to her father.

When I was certain on paper of her existence, I told Bruce, who was excited and welcoming. I wanted him to find a name for her so that we could begin singing her songs as soon as possible. Almost immediately, I began talking to my daughter and welcoming her into this world. I never had an ultrasound to confirm her sex. I just knew I was carrying a girl. My son, the warrior, had come into this world with strength of will and self-confidence. My daughter, the fruit of my deep love for her father, was infusing my soul with tenderness and an overwhelming feeling of oneness with God. In all my meditations, she'd come with a new insight, a new lesson for me. Bruce chose the name Natascia to send a message of peace to Russia, which in those days was still perceived as a potential enemy. Once we settled on her name, I kept asking for inspiration so I could hear her song.

One day, I was reading to Azzurro the old fable of *Snow White and the Seven Dwarfs* by the Brothers Grimm, when I heard her melody. I remembered watching the Italian version of the story when I was a little girl, and recalled the melody of the song the seven dwarves were singing as they went to work in their diamond mine. That night as I went to sleep, I heard the words that were to become her song. *Natascia amore mio, con te tutto il mondo più giocondo sembrera. L'amore è cosa che, ci fa ringiovanir, e ci riempie il cuor di buon umore.* "Natascia my love, with you the whole world will appear a happier place. Love is what makes us forever young and fills our heart with good cheer."

As Natascia grew in my belly, I was searching for materials for my next performance. I had toured with a performance called *Partigiana 1994*, which was the performance I had written and performed while pregnant with Azzurro. I was ready to find the message my daughter had come to share with me. Soon enough, a friend gave me a book from the Italian poet and philosopher Italo Calvino. I'd always loved Calvino; he had lived in Torino, my hometown, and had grown up in the same village where I spent most of my summer vacations when I was little, San Remo. His writing, often described as postmodern, was fantastic yet philosophical in nature. The book I had received, *T Zero*, was a collection of short stories that takes a scientific fact and builds a wonderfully imaginative story around it. Most of my performances up to date had been of an autobiographical nature and at first I doubted I would find any inspiration in the book. That was until I read *Mitosis*, which is the story of a unicellular organism that falls so madly in love with that which is outside itself that it splits into two to experience duality. That, of course, was what had just happened inside my body when Bruce's sperm and my egg collided and became one, then through mitosis split into two, to then become my darling Natascia. So I wrote for her a piece, closely inspired by Calvino's *Mitosis.*[57]

UNDERSTANDING MY LATEST JOURNEY

As I wrote and performed that piece, I began feeling its message of love becoming clearer. My personal interpretation of it, regardless of what the author intended, was that God's first act of creation stemmed from an excruciating, immense, and overwhelming desire to experience Herself by creating duality from the oneness. As in the Hindu tale of Brahman and Atman, God had so much love inside his heart, he wanted to share it, feel it, be part of it. Thus, from one God created two, the apparent duality that at times we seem to experience. This feeling of separation from the source exists simply because we have forgotten that we are one with God. Throughout our lives, we are provided with countless clues to remember our original oneness, so that we may awaken to our true Divine nature and share the bliss of creation.

ONE WITH THE DIVINE—ANATOMY OF LABOR

Every book I have ever read on labor stresses the need for preparation. Unanimously, professionals on both sides of the fence—those who encourage medical solutions to pain-management and those who suggest a more natural approach—preach the importance of informed decisions. We do not know why women feel what they feel during labor and delivery, or why some women feel more, some less. It is speculated that the contractions and their intensity are influenced by a variety of factors including age, life experiences, cultural and familial expectations, and possibly previous traumas, sexual abuse, or painful past experiences. If you read this entire book I hope you have learned to strive to bring more consciousness into your life. Consciousness, self-knowledge, and an understanding of what to expect all contribute to an easier and more joyful experience. Painless childbirth is possible. Not everyone will have a painless experience, yet all your endeavors become possible when one is willing to practice and is dedicated to its fulfillment.

Many women ask me to describe to them what labor feels like, and inevitably I remind them of how hard it is to describe the taste of an artichoke to someone who has never tasted one. Labor often starts with a mild sensation of tightening around your belly. At times there is great pressure in your vagina, and at times most of the sensation is felt in your back around the tailbone, as the baby's head pushes its way out of the birth canal. If the pressure is particularly concentrated on your back it is called back labor. It is more intense, and at times it can be characterized by a steady pressure and pain without the respite between contractions that abdominal labor has. I experienced back labor with my son. By using several positions, like laboring on all fours, having my husband massage and hold pressure on my tailbone, using hot and cold compresses on my back, and soaking in a warm bath, I was able to labor and deliver at home with the help of a midwife and without any drugs. One of the key reasons for my enduring the pressure of back labor was the absence of an alternative to the natural way of coping with the contractions. After all, at home I could not ask for an epidural or any other drugs. Once again, I believe my coping was based on my mindset. Even though the pressure of labor was incredibly intense, I did not have the fear and worry that is associated with pain. I knew why I was feeling the way I was feeling, and I knew the outcome. Also, knowing that women all over the world had endured the same pressure for thousands of years really helped me put my labor in perspective.

Research has shown that "one percent of women [in the United States] report experiencing no pain during childbirth."[58] I was so excited when I heard this. The fact that painless childbirth is a reality was good news. In the United States, there are around four million births each year. So according to the above mentioned study, as many as 40,000 women do experience a painless childbirth! Why not you? Further research also indicates that: "In an analysis of factors thought to influence labor pain, which include fear of pain, confidence, concern about the outcome of labor, frequency of contractions, menstrual pain, and size of the baby, confidence consistently emerged as the most significant predictor of the first stage labor pain."[59] Confidence is what you have been working on throughout this book, affirming your Nine Basic Human Rights to life and your right to fulfill your sacred destiny as a mother. This work has brought you closer to your goal of a painless childbirth.

There are three key words that coincide with the three phases of the first stage of labor: *distraction* in early labor, *concentration* in active labor, and *surrender* during transition. Then we combine purposeful action and concentration during the second stage, the birthing of your baby, followed by exhaustion, elation, and ecstasy in the third stage as you hold the fruit of your loins.

In early labor, you should try to distract yourself from the feeling of the waves of contractions; you should continue your activities as these waves are mild and need very little attention. In active labor, you must concentrate on managing the waves, working hard and, together with your birth coach/partner, using different positions and hypnotic suggestions to ride them. Finally, in transition, you must surrender to the miracle that is at hand and allow the Divine to take over.

EARLY LABOR DISTRACTION

Early labor can start many hours before the actual birth; it can be as short as a few hours or can last days. Often in these hours we get so wrapped up in our desire to hold the baby in our arms that we can easily become discouraged and often exhausted because of its length. I tell all my clients to have an early labor to-do list to fill this time and get their minds engaged in other activities. Early labor projects should combine physical movement with mental, emotional, spiritual, and artistic activities. In the early part of labor we try to distract ourselves from the sensations that our body is feeling. We go on walks, watch a funny movie, listen to music, dance, cook some yummy food, finish up a small project (like a photo album or the crib in the baby's nursery), call on some friends . . . any activity we can conjure up to distract ourselves from looking at the clock and expecting something to happen according to a time schedule. Many women, as soon as they feel the early signs of labor, run to the hospital expecting that once there, something is going to happen. If you go to the hospital too soon, they'll either send you home or try to talk you into being induced. It's best to make peace with the fact that there might be a long day ahead of you. If you have prepared for this, you will have already thought of several activities to do during this wonderful part of labor. This is great time for bonding with your partner and spending one last day as a couple, before you become a triumvirate. I remember spending the early part of my labor with my son, cleaning up my home, creating a birthing altar, choosing music for the birth, and eating foods that reminded me of my home in Italy. With my daughter, I slept during most of early labor, which is another way to distract oneself. In this phase, usually you will dilate from one to three centimeters.

ACTIVE LABOR—CONCENTRATION

In active labor, we use our concentration to manage the increasing waves. Usually in this phase you will dilate from three to seven centimeters. It can last from one to several hours, and you need to use all you have learned to stay focused on what's happening. There are four main activities that I use with my clients in this phase. Alternate between taking a walk, taking a bath, eating and drinking, and resting.

How do we cope with the increasing surges of labor? Many of my clients find it very useful to have their partner remind them where in the minute they are, as a workout coach would do at the gym. Something like, "You're at fifteen seconds, doing well . . . Thirty seconds, you're halfway there . . . Forty-five seconds, you're almost done. That's it . . . almost done, almost done." It's very important that your partner does not announce when he/she thinks the contraction is done and arbitrarily abandon you. Your partner should allow you to let him know when you are ready to be on your own. Partners or your doula should not concentrate on a precision time watch, but rather focus on supporting you physically and emotionally. It's very helpful during this phase for you to continue walking a bit, to change position frequently, to take a warm bath or shower, and to keep hydrated. Studies have shown that "Women who use water immersion during the first stage of labor report significantly less pain than women who do not labor in water."[60]

With the help of hypnosis, I have had several clients who

were able to take little naps during all phases of labor. This is very important, as these phases can last a long time and it's easy to get exhausted. I suggest you either purchase our *Joyful Birth* CD at our Web site www.joyinbirthing.com or find any self-hypnosis CD that will help you nap and relax. Exhaustion is the number one cause for giving up and asking for pain killers once at the hospital. "In the most comprehensive review of literature on the use of hypnosis for pain relief during childbirth, studies involving over eight thousand women were evaluated and it was shown that women who used hypnosis during childbirth rated their pain as less severe than women who did not. The review also concluded that hypnosis reduces the need for pain-relief medication during childbirth."[61]

Hypnosis uses the same tools that religions use to bring people to an altered state of consciousness. All religions have a set of four actions people take in order to arrive at a state of union with the Divine. Some people call this the religious hypnotic process. It involves the following steps:

1. Ritualistic movement. Christians, Muslims, and Jews either genuflect, rock back and forth, or get up and down during their rituals. In yoga, we get into different positions, and Buddhists sit in a lotus position to meditate.

2. Breathing rhythms. Christians recite or sing prayers, as do Muslims and Jews. In yoga and in meditation, we focus on breathing.

3. Eye fascination. Christians, Muslims, and Jews use images in their temples, such as stained glass windows, statues, paintings, or laced sculptural structures. Yoga and Buddhists use mandalas, statues, candles, etc.

4. Hearing stimulation. Once again, Christians, Muslims, and Jews use chanting and singing. In yoga, we often hear meditative music, and Buddhists often chant.

All these actions are similar to the hypnotist's methods used to induce a state of total relaxation and influence. Author and doula Penny Simkin, in her years of practice, has noticed the common denominators among women who manage labor well. In her book, *The Birth Partner,* she explains the three characteristics common among women who cope well:

1. They are able to *relax* during and/or between contractions. In early labor, relaxation *during* contractions is a realistic and desirable goal; later in labor, however, many women cope much better if they don't try to relax during contractions. They feel better if they move or vocalize during the contractions, or even tense parts of their bodies. It is vital, however, that they relax *between* contractions.
2. The use of *rhythm* characterizes their coping style.
3. They find and use *rituals,* that is, the repeated use of personally meaningful rhythmic activities with every contraction.

Now let's combine Ms. Simkin's observation with the religious rituals we mentioned above. As the contraction comes on, it's best to use a ritualistic movement to cope with the wave. It could be hanging on in a slow dance with your partner, sitting on a birthing ball, or any other position you have hopefully learned during your childbirth education class. We couple that with rhythmic breathing—slow, long breaths that envelop and surround your baby. Then you are encouraged to vocalize; I prefer either the *Ahhh* chant or using words like *open, open, open,* and *yes.* When we say *yes,* the universe seems to flood our body with pleasure. Find what works for you and tell your coach. Finally, we use visual images to help us cope. We can visualize our baby working as hard as we are, or we can take ourselves into a safe place where we have experienced serenity and peace. Some of us like to visualize the parts of our body that are working hard, so we can help them open up and hug our baby out.

By using the same methods we have been taught since we were little to worship God, we can embrace our Divine powers and bring our child into this world with the help of the entire universe. Once again, the four stages of inducing what hypnotists call the alpha state (the most transcendent mental state) are the following:

1. Ritual—find a position to go to as you feel the emerging of the wave.
2. Breathe—breathe deeply and use long breaths.
3. Sound—vocalize *Ahhh. Yes. Open.*
4. Visualize—use images that remind you of the baby or those that will give you a sense of peace and serenity.

For example: As the contraction surges, find a position, breathe deeply, vocalize the sound of creation, *Ahhhh,* and visualize your cervix opening up.

TRANSITION—SURRENDER

Transition is by far the most intense of the phases, yet the most welcomed because we know we are close to holding the baby in our arms. In transition, you will usually be dilated between seven to ten centimeters and will become ready to hug your baby out. I have seen transitions that lasted as little as a few minutes and others that lasted a bit longer. Nevertheless, time is only a perception, so it is best not to look at the clock and expect any result based on how much time has passed. In transition, your only requirement is surrender. Your partner best spends his/her time reminding you of the time in between contractions so that you focus on the resting period and not on the intensity of the surges. Take advantage of this time and relax completely. Even close your eyes and try to rest. Many women cannot lie down during transition, but relaxing does not have to be in a reclining position. We can use our partners and doulas to hold our body as we let go and relax in their steady arms. Often, I will coach a woman to breathe deeply and say "Yes" and "Ahhh" as she exhales; this declaration of surrender works to oppose her desire to tense up, fight against the contractions, and say "Oh no!" Here, we remind her often of the outcome, the baby that is working hard to come into this world, and we even address the baby directly with words of encouragement and compassion for all the work that he is doing. It's important to keep the mother focused on the baby; there is nothing a mother will not do for her child if she can envision him working and trying hard. Many of you who have gone through this phase might be furrowing your eyebrows and thinking that as you recall it, it is simply impossible to surrender at this stage. Yet surrender is what is required. By now, you have distracted yourself from the contractions, and then managed and concentrated on them enough to know how to surrender to them. Now it's time to let them take over your body, yielding into them one at a time.

Usually, when clients say, "I can't take it any longer," it indicates that the baby is very close to coming. Very often, women in transition want to give up. They lose hope and courage, as transition resembles the eleventh hour of faith, when all seems lost and we question if God is ever going to come and help. At this juncture, we ask that the midwife, nurse, or physician check the cervix. We often find out that it is dilated to seven or more centimeters (complete dilation is ten centimeters) and the delivery is around the corner. At the news, we rejoice and renew our confidence in the natural state of things. Think about how often you have fretted for some outcome until the proverbial eleventh hour, and then it all got resolved. In labor, this phase is your eleventh hour. This is the time to gather your strength and forge forward. What a great time to practice surrender. We no longer worry and no longer fear. We totally surrender to the beauty that birth is.

I encourage you to surrender to your bodily sensations and take charge of the work that is at hand, visualizing each contraction opening up your cervix more and more. The more you imagine your baby working hard, the more you'll be willing to stick with it and help him through that door.

Yes, you still will try do to the four rituals you did during active labor, but if you truly surrender and let your body do its work, you will probably arrive at the "hugging your baby out" phase much faster. Surrendering is activating your Divine powers. We surrender when we are no longer in control of what is happening and give it all up to our Higher Power. The Mother is there to help; all we have to do is let go and let God. During transition, you will be asked by your care provider, doula, or nurse to alert them if you feel rectal pressure or the desire to push.

HUGGING YOUR BABY OUT

After transition, you will experience a time when contractions spread out again. They generally move to about five minutes apart, but they may stop completely. It's Mother Nature's way to give you a break so that you may gather your energy to hug your baby out. Once the baby passes through the cervix, the uterus needs to snuggle up against the baby, thus I call it hugging the baby out. Some women get the urge to push right away, and their bodies simply involuntarily bear down as if they need to immediately have a bowel movement. Other women don't feel this urge right away as the baby labors down the birth canal. Research has shown that women can benefit from laboring the baby down, especially when the baby's head is still high or not aligned well to the mother's pelvis.[62] Laboring down[63] will lead to a longer second stage than a more active, directed pushing, but it's not as exhausting. Coaching during the hugging phase has been shown to make little difference in the outcome of the birth. Thus a woman who follows her instinctual urges versus holding her breath and pushing for the count of ten will experience fewer medical interventions, such as episiotomy, lacerations, or the use of the vacuum or forceps.[64]

Pay attention to your body: push when your body tells you to push and breathe when your body tells you to breathe. Once again, you know better than anyone who is there to help. Your body was designed for this. At times, and especially in the hospital, you may hear comments like, "Come on, push harder, we need to get this baby out!" Pushing is not a race, and there really is no rush unless the baby is compromised somehow. So make sure your support team asks if the baby is OK and, once reassured, they can whisper gently in your ear, "Everything is OK, listen to your body."

Most women find that it's most comfortable to hold their breath while they push, but this can cut the oxygen going to the baby. This being said, I have seen that some women push more effectively when they hold their breath. So try both ways and go with what feels better. Don't worry if you feel like you're not doing a good job; the baby is on her way and your body will go naturally toward what's best for both of you. Of course, all this works best if your birth is drug-free. If you had to have an epidural, pushing will be more difficult as you may not feel your lower body at all and may have no urge to push.

In this case, allow your team to coach you gently. But again, stress to them that you are in no hurry and that you don't mind the baby laboring down on her own and taking the time she needs to come out. During homebirths, women usually grunt during this phase and tend to do it in six-second intervals instead of the ten-second intervals the hospital suggests.

Most women find relief once they start hugging their baby out; they can actively participate with a specific activity, instead of simply managing a wave. Others experience the greatest intensity at this stage. It's important to keep in mind that the baby is working as hard as you are and that holding him in your arms is right around the corner. Babies go through a peek-a-boo dance where their head peeks out with every hug and then retracts back in when you rest. This can feel frustrating as you get impatient to have your baby on your bosom. I encourage you to touch your baby's head as soon as possible. This will inspire you and help you connect with your child even more. If you're at the hospital, this is also a good deterrent for enthusiastic meddling hands ready to give an episiotomy because, in essence, you are "infecting" the area that has been sterilized.

Changing positions during pushing is extremely important. One squat is worth ten times a supine push, and changes in position can also help decrease the likelihood of tearing. Changing position helps change the angle of your pelvis so that your baby can wiggle her way out, clear the pubic bone, and slide through your pelvis and birth canal.

1. Side-Lying—This is a great position to save energy as well as rotate a baby whose head is either posterior (OP) or transverse (OT).[65] Often after a particularly long labor, I like to start with this position to help the mother rest for a while. Remember, your body will tell you what feels

right, but if you have been in a position for a while and the baby is not peeking through, the more you change position the more you'll help the baby rotate in the right direction.

2. Hands & Knees or All Fours—I love this position because it relieves all the weight from your back and legs. This is one of the best positions to slow a fast second stage, rotate a baby, and reduce tearing. Use this position if you have been stuck at a certain dilation, or if you have been told you have a little cervical lip and there is the risk of a swollen cervix. In this case, go on a chest/knee position with your rear sticking up and your shoulders collapsed on the bed or floor. This can cause the baby's head to temporarily disengage from the cervix and he can hopefully reposition himself.

3. Squatting—Most cultures have used this technique for centuries and for a good reason: this allows gravity to do a lot of the work for you and with you. At times, women are so tired they can't believe they'll have the energy to squat, but simply standing on your feet during the hugging phase will help a great deal. When the urge to hug your baby comes, your body will automatically bend your knees and squat as deep and shallow as you need to be. I have seen many women who apparently failed to progress while supine stand up and deliver their child after a few minutes of hugging their babies this way. This is not a great position if the baby is OP or OT since you should encourage your baby to rotate first.

4. Pushing while on the toilet—This position is best early on since the toilet is a natural place to let go. Also, it's comfortable to sit down without having anything pushing against your vagina. It's not a good position for fast

labor or if you have a strong urge to push as soon as you're ten centimeters dilated.

Bear in mind that if you get an epidural, you will be limited in the positions you can use in the second stage. Unless they turn the epidural off and you feel you can hold your weight, it's unlikely you'll be able to stand or squat. On the other hand, you can still lie on your side and possibly go on all fours. The worst position is indeed a total or partial supine position, lying flat on your back.

I know by now some of you have heard of the ring of fire, the term used to describe crowning, when your baby's head no longer goes in and out but remains stuck at the mouth of your opening, stretching further the passage. Once again, Mother Nature provides relief; the baby's head pressure cuts off the circulation and numbs the surrounding tissues. By no means are you not going to feel it, but it will be a duller sensation than you might think. Just hug that baby through the ring as a lion tamer would incite the lion to spring forth, and remind yourself you are so very close. Finally, the baby's head is delivered and, with a little bit more effort, so is the rest of her body. And here's the miracle. The strong sensations you have experienced thus far ARE ALL GONE. The baby's umbilical cord will still be attached to the placenta, but there should be enough slack for the baby to be put on your chest.

THIRD STAGE—BONDING WITH YOUR CHILD
AND DELIVERING THE PLACENTA

At times this very important stage of the delivery process is either misunderstood, not taken into great consideration, or even brushed off quickly as not as important. Even after a beautiful natural birth at the hospital, I have seen all medical interventions brought back onto this stage. Sarah Buckley, MD, says, "At the time when Mother Nature prescribes awe and ecstasy, we have injections, examinations, and clamping and pulling on the cord. Instead of body heat and skin to skin contact, we have separation and wrapping. Where time should stand still for those eternal moments of first contact, as mother and baby fall deeply in love, we have haste to deliver the placenta and clean up for the next 'case.'"[66]

The moment in which mom and child encounter each other is as important if not more important than all phases of the labor and delivery. As you are looking deeply into your baby's eyes you will discover what love is all over again. Don't expect your baby to breastfeed right away, as most babies need to rest a bit, up to sixty minutes after birth, before they even begin to root for your breast. For the most part, I have seen them simply stare in awe and love at their mom, gently exploring the new world they have come in contact with. This is a great time for you and your partner to come together and once more welcome your baby. It is sometimes necessary to remind doctors and nurses to keep their exchanges down to a whisper as we don't want to distract the baby's ears with unfamiliar sounds. She revels at your voice, and she is eager to listen to her song. If by any chance she needs to be cared for away from you, ask your partner to follow her and talk to her incessantly, explaining all that it is done to her, and reassuring her that she is safe and well cared for. Ask your caregiver to wait until the cord stops pulsating before it is cut; this is to ensure that the baby is still getting blood supply of oxygen at the time of birth, in case she does not breathe on her own immediately.

After your baby is out, your uterus will continue to contract as it begins to work its way back to normal size. As the uterus shrinks, the placenta becomes detached from the uterine wall and is forced down toward the cervix and out the birth canal. It is best to wait for the placenta to deliver naturally than to pull it out. This delivery can take up to one hour.

The first two hours of a baby's life are extremely important; mom and baby should have skin to skin contact and should be allowed to interact without interruptions. The baby does not need to be weighed, measured, or otherwise evaluated if she breathes normally and has a healthy pink color. Most required tests, like the Apgar score, can be performed on the mother's belly. I personally am not too fond of bathing the baby either. Often at the hospital, the baby is bathed and then placed under the warmer because his temperature has plummeted due to the bath. Babies are not dirty, and the mother and child need to smell each other. Now that the baby is in your arms, you will be able to feel the oneness with the creator.

I Am a Drop of the Ocean

I am a drop of the ocean. Place me under a microscope and see that I contain all that the ocean is in its entirety. I am one individual drop. The one who might reach the farthest as I wash ashore. The one who might splash on the hand of a child frolicking at the beach. The one who might touch the sky on the fin of a dolphin. I am simply a drop, but I have within me the power of the tsunami, the ability to transport sustenance and commerce, the privilege of providing fun and joy.

I am a drop of the ocean. And I can be transformed from ocean drop to rain drop. To water the soil and become plant. To rush with the river Nile and cascade in the Niagara Falls. To quench your thirst and become body.

To be blessed and become holy. I am just a drop of the ocean.

But the power of the ocean is within me, and God is within me.

All that I desire is within me, it is me, thus no longer a desire but a reality manifest. I am a drop of the ocean and I am one with you.

WISDOM

A word of wisdom: not all births are the same, and not all women progress at the same level or time. I have had clients who said they couldn't take it anymore when they were dilated three or four centimeters, and others who never showed great distress even at eight and nine centimeters of dilation. The more you prepare yourself to manage one minute at a time, letting go of what will happen next, what you have heard from friends about labor, and what you fear, the more you will be able to handle your labor. Yet, we cannot exclude the possibility that there are physical reasons for painful labor, such as the baby's position or your body's structure.

Pain is something that happens when there is something wrong or unnatural, like an illness or a broken leg. What you are experiencing are the sensations that all women have during childbirth, and the outcome is a happy, lovely baby suckling at your breasts. So, if something goes wrong, like the baby's position, then I encourage you to make informed decisions on the way to implementing a solution. Whether you need some help or medication or even a Cesarean birth, do it from a painless state of being—that is, guilt-free, rancor-free, and resentment-free. All that happens is perfect. We might not understand it at first, but we embrace it as a life lesson that was given to us for a specific, sacred purpose.

During labor, some clients choose to pray. At times, prayers have been seen as actions we take in desperate situations, thus some of us would rather not pray during labor, for we feel that if we do, it is because we are projecting that something has gone wrong or will go wrong. Still, I love to bring God in every action and situation in my life, both dire and happy, for in my prayer I declare how grateful I am. I trust that the outcome I desire is already being manifested here and now.

My Painless Labor and Delivery

Once I had given birth to my son, naturally and at home without the help of any painkillers, I was determined to be in control of the process the next time around. I wanted my experience to be painless. Part of the discomfort I had experienced in my first birth was largely due to fear. I feared the pressure would never end. I feared I was not going to be able to stand it, and I feared my body wouldn't cooperate. In the commotion and excitement, no one had reminded me this was a natural process. No one had whispered in my ears, "Take it one minute at a time."

For my second birth, things were going to be different. I began a regimen of meditation. I visualized the birth step by step and was determined to communicate with my body and tell it to open up at will. It was December 3, 1984. I had a wonderful day, eating my favorite Italian antipasto and nesting at home in preparation for the birth. My mom had come over from Italy and was very worried about me having the baby at home. After all, she had both my brother and me at the hospital, and had had terrible and painful experiences. I realized I had to let go of her fears and her memories, which were still embedded in my consciousness. I didn't allow her worry to enter my space. If any negative thought would rise into my soul, I'd offer it to the Divine Mother to take it away.

I went to bed and slept until midnight; suddenly I woke up and felt wetness between my legs. I turned and whispered into my husband's ear, "It's time, get ready."

The contractions began promptly and followed a specific rhythm. While Bruce called the midwife, I got up and sat on my knees in front of the heater, as it was winter and I was cold. I began to chant *Aaaaaaaaahhhhhhhhhhh*. At each contraction, I would fill up my lungs and allow the sound to come from deep within. I envisioned each breath enveloping my girl with loving arms of fresh air. The sound of my voice relaxed me. I had prepared some music and began tuning inwardly in deep meditation. The waves were coming stronger and stronger. I was anticipating them and riding them with excitement and joy. Nina, my midwife, told my husband to call her back when the contractions were five minutes apart. I let him handle all the logistics; I was determined to be in my special world.

Resting for five minutes and riding the wave for one minute, I was in active labor, so I asked my mother to prepare me a bath. My husband washed the tub thoroughly, and I soaked in the warm water. Nina arrived along with her assistants who had come to see my latest performance. I was going to have a full house.

Shortly after I got in the tub, Nina came into the bathroom and smiled at me. She told me everyone was excited and ready to experience a painless birth. Her confidence raised mine. I stayed in the tub for a while and then felt the need to relieve myself. I remember being on the toilet while my husband, munching on toast, was recording my progress and taping me. *Ahhhhhhhh*—this sound transported me into a new, wondrous world. I imagined my uterus an extension of my arms hugging my baby girl, gently helping her slide down the canal.

I announced I was ready to give birth. Nina asked permission to check my dilation and she carefully and ever so gently checked my status with a flash light, avoiding turning on bright lights. "You have three centimeters to go," she whispered, respecting the sacred space I had entered.

I asked for everyone to leave my bedroom and went under the covers in a fetal position. I closed my eyes and began to visualize my cervix and firmly asked it to open one centimeter with each contraction. Transition set in. I was riding the waves every minute for more than a minute. When the next wave would arrive, strong and powerful, I was ready to ride it, prepared with my surfing board *Ahhhh-hhh,* and my mantra "Open up." At each restful moment, I would visualize imaginary hands tugging at the lips of my cervix. *Ahhhhhhhh.* "One more centimeter," I'd say to my cervix. "Let's do it." *Ahhhhh.*

Three contractions later, I called Nina into my room. "I am ready." She asked permission to check again and, with a smile on my face, I said, "Go ahead, but as soon as you're finished, I'm going to hug my little girl out!" "Yes, you are ten centimeters, completely effaced, and your baby is ready to come."

I remained in a fetal position, allowing my body to go completely limp and loose. I requested the room as dark as possible, so more candles were added around where Nina was working. Mom came over to my side and held my hand. She was crying. I looked up at her and said "Don't worry, Mom, everything will be all right!" I closed my eyes again and simply opened my legs and pushed. I did not hold my breath; it didn't feel like the right thing to do. I simply changed breathing patterns and allowed my body to take over without instructions.

Mother Nature's arms surrounded my womb and we hugged my sweet girl out. In a short ten minutes, Natascia's head popped out. I rested while Nina took the umbilical cord off that had wrapped itself around her neck. I reached and touched my daughter's head. One more celestial hug and my baby was out. Bruce caught our lovely girl as she briskly slipped out of my birth canal. They placed her on my chest and together with my mom we sang her song. "Natascia amore mio, con te tutto il mondo più giocondo sembrerà!"

I had asked not to have my daughter cleaned up, for I believe the vernix was created as the ultimate moisturizer. I massaged it into her skin, delineating for her the confines between her body and the outside world. "Here are your hands, my little one. These are your feet." She laid sweetly there for a while, then began her journey for my breast. She latched on immediately and I continued to sing her song while massaging her. Everyone left us alone, as they went to the kitchen for a cup of tea and some cookies.

There we were, she and I, looking into each other's eyes. Teacher and eager student, the mirror as well as the face in it. One and two, and yet one again with the universe. Love for my child I knew and had experienced, love for my daughter I was just discovering—the intimacy we shared, the Divine connection. I saw in her eyes my grandchildren, I saw in her the creative legacy passed down from mother to daughter. Rumi's words came to mind, "When I am with you, we stay up all night. When you're not here, I can't go to sleep. Praise God for these two insomnias! And the difference between them."

The birth had been joyful and painless. Our son (two years old) had woken up just in time. He walked into the bedroom, rubbing his eyes with his little fists. "Here is your baby sister," his father showed him. His eyes became big for a moment; he said, "Sista." He came over, kissed me ever so sweetly, and went right back to bed.

I got up and took a shower while Mom and Bruce cleaned and prepared my bed. Bruce and I lay down with our new bundle of joy, who fed all night long while we rested. Natascia was born at 3:45 a.m. on December 4, 1984, in my home in Marina Del Rey in the same bedroom I still sleep in. If I can do it, so can you!

THE NINE BASIC HUMAN RIGHTS

Close your eyes and go to your heart center. Look at all that you have learned thus far about yourself, about your negative core beliefs, about your deeply rooted fears and your limitations, and see it from your loving heart as a compassionate witness with no shame or blame. Become willing and fully able to let go of those false judgments about yourself and about what is coming. Embrace the truth that you are the mother that God created you to be, perfect in every way, yet not striving or wanting to be perfect. Simply know that the perfection of God is within you and that there are no mistakes in the eyes of the Divine. That all that happens has a good reason, a God reason, and that there is no punishment or reward.

Feel the power rising from your lower chakra in your perineum. Feel the warmth that surrounds your belly and your baby who sits between the second and third chakra. Empower your child with his right to take action in the birthing experience from a place of self-confidence. Allow the love to explode and flood from your heart onto every fiber of your being. Feel the beauty that you are and that is still growing within you and all around you. Feel the energy that surrounds your throat, giving you the voice of strength and self-assertiveness. Know that you have the knowledge of all our ancestors channeling through you. Feel worthy of the miracle that is birth, worthy of being the vessel through which the Divine expresses itself. Know and embody your oneness with the Divine. See the energy float gently upward and once again downward without obstacles, clearing the way, freeing the passage from God through your baby into this world. Feel it, see it, accept it, agree with it, become one with it, and be grateful for it.

A Prayer

I have the right to have a painless childbirth; I have the right to be here to live and thrive in this world. I have the right to feel my feelings and express them safely. I have the right to want my desires fulfilled. I have the right to act according to my knowledge, my beliefs, and my dreams. I have the right to love and be loved, for God loves all His children. I love myself and my child unconditionally. I have the right to speak and hear the truth. I have the right to see and be seen. I have the right to know all I need to know to bring forth my child joyfully, naturally, and painlessly. I have the right to Divine power, for I am a vessel of Mother/Father/God. I have the right to be one with the miraculous. There is no separation between me and the Divine; I am one with IT. Being grateful that all my desires are already here, manifested in the now, I release them into the universe, knowing they'll come back fulfilled. And so it is. Amen.

10

the art of letting go

I surrender my birth over to the care of the Divine Mother. I let go of all my expectations, my plans, and even my desires. Thy will be done. As I do this, I birth a human being who is unencumbered by fear. My highest and best unfold when I learn to let go and let God. I am eternally immersed in God, and God is eternally immersed in me. I enter the sacred space of nurturer and sustainer of my child, and the triumphant sound of gratitude rings through my baby's voice, my action, and state of being. So be it. Amen.

The concept of letting go may seem easy at first, yet it is probably one of the most challenging lessons in a person's life. There are three categories of letting go: 1) physical, 2) psychological, and 3) spiritual. Even though these categories are interrelated, to simplify the process we will relate to them as separate.

We have all learned the difficulty of letting go of some material possession. We had to let go of a house we really liked, clothes we just couldn't fit into anymore, a favorite object. When we ended a relationship, we had to let go of the physical touch we were used to. Big or small, letting go was not easy. At times, it left us feeling empty, lonely, and sad. Yet, we have also let go of unwanted pounds and let go of clutter, and we felt lifted by the experience. When we get close to the time our child joins us in our home, we experience the nesting instinct that instinctively makes us go around and rearrange our living quarters, letting go of the way things were around the house. We are making room for our bundle of joy to join us and have his rightful place next to us.

Throughout this book we have worked extensively at psychologically letting go of people, places, and things that no longer serve us. The process, although a bit painful, has also turned out to be refreshing and renewing. Logically, we understood the need we have to let go of anger, fear, rancor, and resentment, and we have learned the tools to check ourselves in our daily lives for evidence of those feelings resurfacing, so that we may understand them and bring love and compassion to them in order to exorcize them. When we allow ourselves to let go of our need to be perfect and we allow others the same privilege, we set ourselves up for success.

Letting go at the physical and psychological levels has given us freedom. After all, when we hold tightly to something, it becomes that which runs our lives more than the other way around. I've often heard successful people tell me that if we go to a job interview not "needing" the job, we are more likely to get it. Needing the job, money, object, or person enslaves us to the erroneous concept that we cannot live without it. On the other hand, when we enter any situation not needing it, we enter as free individuals whose emotional state cannot be altered by that which is outside of them. Dr. Beckweth once said, "When you wake up in the morning, be a thermostat, not a thermometer."[67] What he meant was that a thermometer changes its state according to outside influences, and a thermostat changes the environment that surrounds it by raising or lowering the temperature according to its programming.

Which brings us to letting go spiritually. If the thermostat has been programmed only by us, it will have within it our human characteristics and personality. After all this work, we might certainly be better than we were, but by all means we still have a long way to go. So why not let the Mastermind of the Divine do the programming. This in essence is what the dictum *Let go and let God* really means.

In chapter eight, you defined your Higher Power and by its definition, God/the universe/Mother Nature, whatever you want to call it, it will have perfect and Divine qualities. Thus, if you let it do the programming, your temperature will be perfect. Letting go and letting God means that we openly declare that God, our Higher Power, is a stronger and greater source of power than we are, and that once we have done our best, it is up to our Higher Power to take over. How do we do this? How does one let go and let God? While my son and I were editing this book, he would often make the following comment, "Mom, it seems so easy to simply state a desire and it is so, but in reality giving our lives over to the care of God is not that easy. What are the practical steps; how do I let go?"

Letting go is a daily and sometimes hourly reprieve. When we find ourselves in a state of anxiety, in fear, or when we cannot stop the chatter in our mind, we need to make an effort to literally announce, "I let go of all this that is taking my serenity away. Please God take it and do with it what you will. All is good, all is God." The simple act of declaring our resolve not to dwell on that which does not serve us and affirming our desire to let a power greater than ourselves take it from us, will eventually get you to a state of serenity. It is simple but not easy.

In the next four to six weeks it is the time to practice patience and the art of letting go of your expectations, of your attachment to how, when, and where you will have this baby. Homebirths have gone to the hospital and hospital births have occurred at home. Both situations may seem scary, but in perfect design there are no mistakes.

BABIES ARE NOT PUNCTUAL

Waiting for the big moment to arrive deserves its own special chapter. Your pregnancy can go quickly or drag on and on. The last few weeks can feel like the longest in your life. Some women are so "done" with pregnancy by this time that they are ready to do anything to get the baby out, even induce or schedule a Cesarean birth.

Your baby will come when it is his time to come. If you really think about it, once he's born, are you going to rush him? "Come on, can't you eat faster? Grow faster! Crawl faster!" You will be patient and loving. You will wait for him as he slowly takes his first step. Why should birth be any different? Your child is preparing to come into this world, and that's a big job. Enjoy these last few days. Once your child is born, the two of you will be on a slow but sure path of separation. When birth is past its due date, you will start hearing about natural and medical methods of induction. Actually, many doctors will talk about induction or even propose it as early as thirty-nine weeks, but beware of such proposals. Asking the right questions will help you make informed decisions.

BISHOP SCORE

This month, you must be prepared for some of the language you will hear at your doctor's office. Recently, as a result of the dramatic rise in the number of artificially induced labors, there have been several articles published on the risks of induction. Some doctors are induction-happy; they like to schedule their lives. It's a tough job to always be on call, and strictly from that point of view, if they can schedule their lives better, they will. Furthermore, until recently, most doctors truly believed that artificial induction was acceptable. Looking at the high rate of Cesareans, we now know that failed inductions stand as one of the most common reasons for such a consequence. Still, if a doctor sees that you're getting impatient toward the end of your pregnancy, he might suggest an induction. Most doctors really believe that inducing is not harming the child. Nevertheless, inducing is indeed opening the door to possible complications. Your baby might not like Pitocin, and his heart rate may fall, resulting in an emergency Cesarean birth. You might not be able to take the strength of the contractions and so will ask for an epidural, which often opens the door for more medical interventions.

Recently, at a conference with a group of osteopathic doctors,[68] I learned that Pitocin-induced contractions for a prolonged time can severely interfere with the musculoskeletal system of the baby. "Birth often results in harmful structural changes. The likelihood of trouble increases when the labor and delivery is prolonged or augmented by Pitocin or when forceps or vacuum extractions are necessary."[69]

If your care provider seems impatient, be informed and arm yourself with the following facts. To obtain a successful induction, your Bishop Score should be greater than nine.[70] Ask for the specifics of your baby's position, the consistency of your cervix, the degree of effacement, dilation, and your baby's station (which indicates where your baby's head is at the time of the vaginal exam). When you add all the values, you should have a Bishop Score of nine to have a successful induction. Be sure to ask your caregiver for your Bishop Score.

Cervix	Score			
	0	1	2	3
Position	Posterior	Midposition	Anterior	—
Consistency	Firm	Medium	Soft	—
Effacement (%)	0–30	40–50	60–70	>80
Dilation (cm)	Closed	1–2	3–4	>5
Station	−3	−2	−1	+1, +2

You might also be induced on the basis of not enough amniotic fluids. In the last few weeks of pregnancy, your amniotic fluids and your baby's heartbeat will likely be checked often. It's always best to ask for specifics. For example, you may be told, "Your fluids are low," as one of the reasons why you should be induced. Know that if your fluids are at five centimeters or more and the baby's heartbeat is fine, all is well. If your fluids are barely less than five (such as 4.9), you might just need a glass of water. If they're four or less, you must be induced. Get a second opinion on your fluid levels at the hospital. Often, a new, inexperienced technician will miscalculate, and sometimes the machines at a doctor's office are not as accurate as those at the hospital. If you're sent to the hospital for low fluids, ask, "Is this an emergency, or do I have some time?" If you've been given time enough to go home and get your bags, this is not an emergency, so you may consider the following:

- Before you go to the hospital, have a good meal. Once you get there, they will not feed you until the baby comes. This will only take thirty minutes, but it will make a huge difference in your energy level during the induction.
- Prepare yourself emotionally; being induced is not the end of the world. Many of my clients have successfully had a drug-free birth even when induced. Call your doula or your support team; they will help. Take a moment and sit still; if you know how to meditate, this is a great time to do so. Center and tell yourself everything will be OK. Rushing to the hospital will get you off center. Low amniotic levels are usually not a terrible emergency. Remember, there is always enough time to come back to center and talk to your baby.
- Once you are at the hospital, ask them to re-measure the levels. Ask for the numbers, and if your levels are five or more centimeters, ask if you can leave. You may be asked to go in and check your levels often, which is a good idea, be available for weekly neonatal stress tests (where your baby's heartbeat will be checked and monitored), and possibly a few more ultrasounds. Collaborate with your care providers; they are there to help. Even if it's annoying to go and get checked every two or three days, take this time to communicate with your child. As you listen to her heartbeat, ask your baby to tell you if there's anything in the way of her entrance into this world.

If you're going to leave the hospital, call your doctor and tell him/her you'd like a little more time to see if the baby comes naturally. At this time, I would advise acupuncture or a chiropractic visit to try natural induction. Hypnosis really helps to find out if there are any fears left that stand in the way of this birth, and to relax and accept the outcome.

Often, it's a real struggle to leave the hospital once you've entered following doctor's orders. Choose your battles wisely; any day is a good day for a stress-free birth. If you decide to stay and begin the induction, ask to manage the rate at which the Pitocin is administered, and together with your birthing team you can embrace the contractions one at a time. Usually nurses will come every fifteen to twenty minutes and automatically raise the Pitocin levels without even asking you. Gently express your desire to manage the contractions and ask the nurse to ask you before she raises the level. You are not to follow a time schedule that was established by the hospital procedures or the medical books; as long as your baby is doing well and you are progressing, there's no need to follow any schedule. As suggested earlier, make friends with the nurse right away. Ask her about her birth, her children, the weather, anything. Remember, give love and you will receive love in return.

Gently manage your Pitocin-induced contractions one at a time, visualizing your cervix opening up. If your Bishop Score is low, the doctor might suggest cervadil (prostaglandin gel that's placed within or near the cervix to ripen it). The application of the gel may be repeated once after twelve hours. At times, just the gel alone will start contractions. The advantage of using this method is that the gel comes in a coil with a string attached to it, and if you or your baby experiences any negative side effects, the gel can be removed. Beware of doctors who suggest Cytotec as a ripening or labor-inducing agent. The drug Cytotec is NOT approved by the FDA for this use and it is very controversial. If your doctor or midwife tells you she uses Cytotec, please go on the Web and inform yourself. Then make a decision whether you want to have it used on you or not. Remember, there are other medicines out there to induce labor. You have a choice. Visit www.motherfriendly.org, The Coalition for Improving Maternity Services (CIMS), and read their research on the hazards of induction.

NATURAL INDUCTION METHODS

If your doctor has scheduled an induction date, please discuss these methods with your care provider.

- Relaxation techniques. Tension works against labor. Use visual imagery. Try hypnosis, as it is known to work wonders with tension. By relaxing deeply and completely, you may be surprised to find yourself in labor. A good cry also relieves tension; get a tearjerker movie and let it rip.
- Sex. Sex has long been a method of inducing labor. The prostaglandin in semen and orgasm can stimulate contractions. While some of my clients do not feel like having sex in the last month of their pregnancy, it sure beats a Cesarean birth or medical induction! It will not harm the baby, and female orgasm can open the cervix up to two centimeters. If you really are not in the mood, try inserting his sperm as close to the cervix as possible.
- Nipple stimulation. Nipple stimulation can successfully induce labor. Uterine hyper-stimulation may be avoided by following a protocol. Ask your care provider for a specific technique.
- Exercise. Walking, swinging on a swing, and exercise in general helps contract the uterus.

- Bumpy car ride. A bumpy car ride may sound like an old wives' tale, but if the baby is not in a good position, sitting and relaxing while the car moves over bumps can help reposition the baby and facilitate the head engagement.

- Enemas. Enemas cause the bowels to contract and could stimulate the uterus to contract, which will open and efface the cervix. Use with caution.

- Use of herbs. Several herbs are used by midwives to induce labor or to stimulate contractions. Do NOT take any of these herbs without first conferring with a midwife, physician, and herbalist. Labor-enhancing herbs include red raspberry leaf, evening primrose oil (ripens the cervix), castor oil. If you use castor oil, three teaspoons is about right. Try mixing it with some juice or pour it over a green salad or a tuna salad. A word of caution: castor oil can cause cramps and diarrhea. If you know how you react to strong laxatives, then you can decide whether to use this method of induction.

Try a visit to a chiropractor who specializes in the Webster technique,[71] or to an acupuncturist, and/or a reflexologist. While no official evidence exists regarding acupressure and inducing/stimulating labor, many perinatal specialists, midwives, physicians, childbirth educators, and doulas confirm the relationship between acupressure points and increased uterine contractions. When it comes to natural induction, if your body is not ready, nothing will work.

Pamper yourself, talk to your child. Tell her you are willing to wait until she is ready to come. If you can, take the last two weeks off from work to focus on the sacred event. Remember to laugh: see funny movies, enjoy this time. Please know that it is OK for a baby to come out as late as two weeks after the due date. Ask your care practitioner how he feels about letting you wait a bit longer. Don't rush into things. Let go and let the perfection of nature lead you. One of the angels who came to help me out with this book wrote me this lovely story about how her mom helped her induce labor.

An Unusual Induction Story from Annette

When it comes to induction methods, my mom had a good one. I was two weeks late with my son. She got edgy to get home to her work and family, whom she missed, so one morning she said, "Let's go to the Farmers Market and bump around in the crowd. Getting twenty miles away from the hospital will do it every time." I was skeptical, but went along. Soon after we got to the Farmers Market, I felt the first contraction, but I didn't say a word. This went on for hours as the contractions got more and more intense. We sat down to eat in an open-air place. Soon my mother said, "Are you ready to go to the hospital?" I said, "Why do you ask?" She smiled as she pronounced, "I know my daughter; you can't fool me."

The ride to the hospital forty minutes away in traffic was an adventure, and I insisted on driving. We hung around the hospital walking up and down waiting for the doctor to finally arrive. He told me the same thing I assume he said to all his clients, almost as a hypnotic command, "I'll be back in three hours to deliver your baby." Three hours later, my son was born. I later found out that nearly all my doctor's clients, after arriving at the hospital and getting a visit from him, indeed delivered in three hours.

WILL MY LIFE CHANGE FOREVER?

Once the baby is born, your life will change forever. It will change in so many ways, and until you get there you simply can't be told. The joys, the sorrows, the excitement, the fear, the frustrations—in fact, I think all the adjectives in the world couldn't describe what is in store for you.

We often hear mothers say, "It was difficult at times, but it has been worth it." Yes, it is worth it, the journey is fantastic. Even if this is not your first baby, another one does bring new changes.

I remember asking myself, "What about all the things I wanted to do? Have I lost all hope now?" Hope should never die. Let's make a list of all the things you've wanted to do, but that you haven't had the time, money, or guts to do. Go crazy and be outlandish with the list; it doesn't have anything to do with what you can afford or realistically do right now. The purpose of this list is to write down all of your dreams and desires, from small to out-of-this-world.

Once you are finished with your list, place it somewhere you can see it. Every day, find a creative way to fulfill one of your wishes. For example, if you wished to go to Africa, go down to your local video store and rent movies and documentaries about Africa. Dress yourself up in your favorite African traveling garb, and enjoy the show.

If you always wanted to live in a mansion, go to an open house listed in your local paper. Walk around as if you owned the place; look out one of the windows and pretend you are there alone, looking out of your own window. Indulge yourself in that feeling. The more you feel it, the more you will bring it into manifestation.

Take care of the little wishes too, like calling an old friend you haven't talk to in a long time, or going out for a romantic candlelight dinner with your loved one. Don't wait for him to ask and plan. This is your wish list, so take charge and have fun with it. Make sure to check off all the wishes that are coming through for you. The joy of a wish list increases as you progressively fill it with checkmarks of accomplishments. You are the creator of your own reality. Have fun with it, share it with your husband, and invite him to add his wishes to the list or to make one of his own. Some men are practical, and they'll try to tell you how certain things just don't make any sense. If he starts telling you how this or that on your list cannot be possible, gently tell him that all dreams are possible and writing this list makes you really happy.

PLAN YOUR BABYMOON

The concept of the babymoon was first introduced by childbirth educator and author Sheila Kitzinger. The babymoon is a special time when you and your partner are alone with your new baby. It's a special time for your love to grow, to experience the deepest closeness, and to get to know your baby without the intrusion of the usual responsibilities and social contacts.

Make it your second honeymoon. Plan to spend as much time as you can together, just the three of you, getting to know each other all over again, rejoicing in each other's presence. Plan to turn your bed into an island of love.

Ask family and friends to help you plan your babymoon. Make sure everyone understands you need their help, but you will not and cannot give them your full attention. This is your time, a once-in-a-lifetime chance to get to know your new family. There will be plenty of time for all your family and friends to see the baby and participate in your life. Ask them to come and go gently and softly, so that the three of you can be peaceful and comfortably alone in this magical bonding time.

If you tell people in advance that you will be spending your babymoon at home in peace, they will understand. Ask people to come and help with your other children, but make sure brothers and sisters get in on the babymoon, too. Get an answering service and place a lovely announcement on it with all the important news. "Our baby was born at ____, she/he is ____ pounds, healthy and joyful. Baby, mommy, and daddy are on our babymoon. We'll get in touch as soon as we get back."

Now, fill your refrigerator, fill your cupboards, fill your heart, fill your soul, fill your life with your Higher Power, and get ready for the magic to unfold.

PLANNING AHEAD

During the first few weeks of motherhood, caring for the baby and yourself will take just about all of your time and energy. Planning now can make a world of difference. We have already talked about the babymoon concept, so we have tackled how your partner and support people can help out. Now you are prepared practically, but what about emotionally? I remember when my first child was born, I experienced what I called "opening of the heart," normally referred to as postpartum blues. Yes, even after all this preparation, after all this Divine experience, I felt blue. After all, I had loved my pregnancy; I loved preparing for it, meditating for it, eating for it, and feeling I was in control. I loved the birth and the choices I had made. I was proud of how it went and how close to God, my husband, my child, and my girlfriends I was. But now it was all over. Sure I had a bundle of joy in my arms, sure I loved this baby more than life itself, but I had not prepared myself for the powerlessness over my life I experienced after the birth. I no longer was in charge of when I was going to eat, sleep, rest, be up, and go places. My life was not only changing, it was no longer under my control; Azzurro, my son, was running it. The most useful resource I found was another woman in the same situation;

it seemed she was truly the only one who understood me, who knew and felt what I was going through. Look for a support system right now, a mothers' group you can join with your baby. They will not be surprised when you say, "Sometimes I just want to cry all day." Remember this too shall pass, and make this your mantra during the next twelve weeks. Sometimes these feelings intensify, so pay attention to them and practice self-care.

BABY BLUES OR OPENING OF THE HEART

In my years of practice, I have always made sure to let every mom-to-be know about the phenomenon called the "baby blues." My training taught me that the subject should not only be discussed, but that I should be prepared with informational materials on postpartum depression, and that I should show the partner how to look for signs of depression.

Once, during an appointment with a client, I was going through my spiel on what to expect after the birth when Divine intervention revealed something to me: What if we renamed the baby blues, calling them something closer to their purpose? That would be: opening of the heart.

What really happens in those weeks and months that follow birth? Why are we teary, emotional, and sensitive? I suggest that our hearts open wide when we hold our first true love in our arms. Sure, we have loved a man (or woman, or two) deeply in our lives. Some of us experienced true love for a brother or sister, or for our parents. But as we grew up, our hearts closed up a little bit each and every day.

Our hearts may have closed up for self-preservation after our first breakup, or because we were hurt by a family member, or because a friend (even someone we thought was our best friend) hurt us. We have even shouted to the heavens, "I will never fall in love again!" by way of attempting to lock those doors and throw away the key. Then we allowed our partners in. We may have made a conscious decision to have a child, and in so doing we cracked the doors of our hearts slightly ajar. Yet, when our baby, our angel incarnate, was placed on our bosom, the gates of our heart flew open. We became enchanted with how much we could feel. Of course we cried often; we became emotional and sensitive.

But what people call the blues was in essence a very ancient feeling, one that shocked us and even overwhelmed us. We asked ourselves, "Is it possible we are truly able to love this much? Can we bear it? Do we deserve it? Are we good enough to be mothers? When did we feel like this before? Did we not love our mom as much when we were first born? Did we not cry to be in her arms?"

We wondered if our mothers felt the same as we do right now. We felt a longing to be loved that way again. This opening of the heart sometimes permits hurt feelings from the past to surface, to clamor for our attention. We remember losing our innocence after something hurt us terribly. Our unconscious could no longer hold these buried memories, these secrets. We felt a fog waft over us, mixed with fear and for some even terror. We hoped and prayed those feelings would soon go away and not develop into something more serious. We allowed ourselves some stolen tears, but were careful to control the outcome.

Once I went to visit a client who had just had a Cesarean. Laden with bags full of groceries, I set to making her a vegetarian feast. She had an overactive let down and was producing a lot of milk. As a consequence, her baby spit up a lot. I saw that her baby was very fussy and that she was at the end of her rope. Showing her a few tricks to calm her baby down, I placed the now sleepy bundle in her arms and invited her to sit down in the kitchen and tell me about her birthing experience.

Feeling safe, she proceeded to tell me how lonely she felt, and how having her baby spit up all over everything made her feel inadequate. When she was told that the baby had acid reflux, she concluded that she was doing everything wrong. She asked me to "Please, just listen," for she had so much information swimming in her mind that she just couldn't hold anymore. She began to pour her heart out, tickled by the scent coming from my cooking pots.

Toward the end of the day and after a good meal, she said, "Today I was driving with my boy and thought, 'Maybe I can just drive myself off a cliff and all this would be over.' Mind you," she added with a forced smile, "I'd never do such a thing. But I just thought about it." I asked for her permission to embrace her and whispered, "I think it's time you talk to someone." I explained the opening of the heart concept and asked her to consider making an appointment with a professional. She smiled; someone finally had given her permission to express and feel her feelings.

That evening her husband called, very worried, "Are you sure this is not temporary? This is not what you call the blues?" "No," I responded gently, "this is not the blues. Your wife's heart has opened up! It is wonderful that you can hear her and help her to get the help she needs to explore her feelings." They made an appointment and she was in therapy for nearly nine months.

By allowing her to truly feel and to express what was going on in her mind, she was freed to seek help. Stories from her past had surfaced after childbirth, and they demanded her attention, NOW. Grateful that someone had allowed her to open her heart and clean her emotional house, she learned to enjoy motherhood, breastfeeding, and my Italian cooking.

What if we were to embrace this opening of the heart and rejoice in feeling deeply that which presents itself, permitting this sensation to last as long as it is needed before we close ourselves up again in self-preservation? Yes, some of us will go through a period of depression, but that is precisely nature's wonderful way of saying, "It's time you heal these wounds. Get some help now, and you'll be an even better mother for it!"

"But wait," we say, "there is no time! I have things to do and people to see. I have to be the mother, the protector, the caretaker. I have to be strong for my baby. I cannot fail." Breathe in! There is no failure here. Remember that you are in love: have you forgotten the First Love? Do you not remember daydreaming more than taking care of business? Embrace your feelings, spend time daydreaming with your bundle of joy at your breast.

I suggest that you prepare and organize yourself so that for the first few weeks postpartum you do nothing but live this love. The few weeks that follow the birth should be dedicated to self-care. If you can, go outdoors and breathe deeply God's clean air, ask for help, eat and sleep often, cuddle in bed, and let people care for you. Slow down: it is OK for the dishes to be dirty, the floor unwashed, your e-mail unopened, and the telephone unanswered. Write in your journal, talk to a trusted friend or a professional.[72] Find a postpartum doula or someone who can come and help you, someone who does not need to be entertained or cared for. Knowing what to expect and what steps you can take toward self-care will ensure that once the doors are open, you need not struggle to keep them closed anymore, for you will learn how to create healthy boundaries to protect your open heart.

BRINGING HOME THE BABY

The first twelve weeks of a new baby's life are challenging for both the parents and the baby. When I conduct my postpartum visit at the homes of my clients, I usually find three very tired and frustrated people. Mom and partner have not slept, baby is adjusting, and breastfeeding often is not so natural. The latch on is not something that is innate in either the mother or baby. In the past, we grew up seeing women breastfeed, and as little girls we were privy to the conversations women had about their challenges and the various solutions the women of the village suggested. Today we live in an isolated world. Our mothers, for the most part, were told that breastfeeding was at best vulgar, that only poor and ignorant women did it, for formula was the modern woman's way.

Thank God things have changed radically, yet even those mothers who breastfed their daughters often don't remember much and can be of no practical help if there is a problem. Certainly a mother can support emotionally what her daughter is going through, but if you need a professional, please don't hesitate to ask for help. A breastfeeding problem that might seem huge to you might be fixed in minutes by a professional lactation consultant, or a breastfeeding peer at La Leche League. Please visit my Web site at www.joyinbirthing.com to get an updated list of lactation organizations in the United States, or ask your pediatrician for a referral.

Planning your postpartum period ahead of time is very important. Who will be your support system? Will you hire help? Will you enlist family or friends to help you? Make a list of things you will need once the baby is at home, and when friends and family offer to help, show them the list and ask them to pick out what they would like to do. Making lists gives them choices; you will not feel embarrassed to ask, and it will steer you away from the "Thanks, but I think I'm OK" syndrome.

One of the most successful tools I have found to help parents care for their new baby is Dr. Harvey Karp's DVD *The Happiest Baby on the Block* and his CD of soothing white noise. Dr. Karp explains that babies are born three months before they are fully ready for the world and they benefit from a "4th trimester" of holding, rocking, and nurturing. He teaches parents that all babies are born with a "calming reflex"—a virtual off switch for crying. The DVD shows five ways (called the 5 Ss) that can help any parent "turn the switch off" and become skilled at gently helping calm a fussy baby. What I love about it is that it empowers your partner to become the champion baby calmer, giving him/her some specific tools to jump in and help. I also like to refer to it as the mother pampering tool as it has been shown to help prevent postpartum depression often associated with lack of sleep. The white noise CD is designed to imitate the rich sensory environment of the womb and when played next to the baby it will actually prolong your baby's sleep, lulling her with familiar sounds.

Another very important factor to remember about babies is that they are full-fledged people. Often, when I visit a couple and their newly born baby, I notice that the parents change the baby's diapers, pick him up from the crib, or hand him over to me without asking him permission or telling him what's going on. How would you like it if I just came up to you, took you by the hand, and took you into another room without any explanation? Just because babies don't talk back doesn't mean we don't need to ask their permission or tell them what we are about to do. Besides, talking to your baby immediately and showing her respect is a two-folded gift. First, you will establish a mutual, respectful relationship. Second, as you talk to him, you'll bring him into consciousness. He'll stay awake longer, he'll respond earlier to stimuli, and he'll develop his neurological functions at an early age.

I once acted as the guest expert for a television show on TLC called *Bringing Home Baby*. They called me in to help a family with a thirty-six-hour old baby. The mom was having trouble breastfeeding, and the dad and grandma were in tears in response to the frustration that the new mom was experiencing. What are the infant's needs, beyond those for food, rest, warmth, and hygiene? All parents do show their love and voice their affection to infants, but they often forget to talk to their babies as they would an adult. It is not only loving, but respectful to ask permission and let a child know what is about to happen to them. By telling the baby where they were taking her, letting her know they were about to change her diaper, about to give her to mom to feed, or about to give her a gentle sponge bath, they began seeing amazing results. I showed the dad how to talk to his baby. I taught him how to hold her in a football position and tell her all about the new family she had joined. The baby, for the first time, stayed awake for over three hours in the comfort and safety of her dad's arm, looking around and taking in the wonder of the new world. The mom, dad, and grandma were surprised, and they saw how talking to the child constantly brought the new life over into the conscious world. They understood the need to modify their relationship with their little one and began considering her as another person who had needs, wants, and a great deal of curiosity.

Learn how to play simple games with your newborn. Lock eyes with her and then gently tip your head to the right or left and watch her follow. Another fun game is called the imitation game. Wait for the baby to focus on your face and stick out your tongue at her. Repeat this a few times and allow the child to move her entire body. You'll see that eventually she will imitate you. These games can be very tiring, so don't overdo them. There is a great video called *The Amazing Talents of the Newborn* that can show you how to play with your baby from the very beginning.[73]

Babies love routine. They love to know that things happen at a certain time following a certain ritual. I encourage my clients to read to their infants in the evening at the same time, before they lie down with their precious bundle to go to sleep. Following a routine that the parents and child can hang on to helps manage the tough times ahead. Just as in labor we practiced how to manage the waves of contractions by having a plan of action, so I encourage you to create a plan of action to implement when the baby comes home. Knowing there is a routine to be followed and a specific set of steps to handle any situation that may arise can put the mother and baby's mind at ease.

A simple routine I propose is to divide the day into two twelve-hour segments. Please understand that these are suggestions that need not be taken literally, for caring for a newborn is instinctual and should not be done on a schedule. That being said, research has confirmed that babies like consistency of rituals throughout their day because it provides a greater sense of stability.[74] The first twelve hours will be your baby's daytime, and the second set her nighttime. During the day, establish a specific set of rituals, like waking up and sponge-bathing her. Start the day by telling her, "Good morning, my love," and change her in into some daytime clothes. Then make sure you play with her, talk to her, engage her gaze, put her on her tummy for tummy time, feed her, and cuddle her to sleep. Plan an afternoon outing, even if it's just on your balcony or porch; the fresh air will benefit both of you. Then an afternoon nap for the two of you, and toward the end of the evening a soothing and relaxing bath and baby massage. Then you can announce to the baby that it's bedtime and you put her pajamas on and read her a story while she feeds. The next twelve hours will have a different quality to them, as you will not play with her, not engage her gaze or talk to her, keep the light soft and low, and efficiently feed her in bed next to you as you attempt to sleep yourself.

Knowing what to expect and what is coming every day will give your baby something to hang on to and will train you to be consistent with her. So once she's a toddler it will not be a question of whether it is time to go to sleep, but rather which story does she want you to read before she goes to sleep. For she will have followed a ritual since the day she was born and will be happy to participate in the decision-making that is appropriate for her age, such as which book to read.

Angie's Story

It's Friday, full moon, and Fourth of July weekend. The hospital is crowded with women getting induced before the long weekend, and there are no beds available. Doctors are trying to get as many women delivered as possible so they can have a restful weekend. But not Angie's doctor. He wants her to come into the hospital because she is five centimeters dilated, twelve days past due (second baby), and he's concerned that if her waters break at home, she won't make it to the hospital on time. She has been dilating almost a centimeter every two or three days, but feels no strong contractions. It's a totally painless early labor, so much so she doesn't feel like she's in labor at all. She is admitted at 12:30 p.m. and the doctor breaks her waters at 1:15. I join her at 1:45 and the contractions have already picked up a nice rhythm. We move around in different positions, using the birthing ball and the bed to dance the birthing dance. She goes into a deep state of relaxation following my hypnotic suggestions. She is concentrating and managing each wave spectacularly. By 2:00 p.m. the contractions are one minute apart and strong, and you can see her smiling as she rides them with determination. By 2:30 she is involuntarily pushing. The doctor shows up at 2:37. He checks her and announces she is fully effaced, fully dilated, and the baby is at +2 station. It's time to hug her baby out. Her husband and I each take one foot, resting it on our shoulders, and Angie pushes with all her might. The baby is crowning. By 3:54, her baby is born, a beautiful eight-pound baby. Angie's perineum is intact, and her baby girl is hungry. Total labor time was one hour and twenty-four minutes. Amazing. What a woman, what a birth. Painless; yes, it can be done.

Do Not Believe in Anything I Tell You

Do not believe in anything simply because you have heard it. Do not believe in anything simply because it is spoken and rumored by many. Do not believe in anything simply because it is found written in your religious books. Do not believe in anything merely on the authority of your teachers and elders. Do not believe in traditions because they have been handed down for many generations. But after observation and analysis, when you find that anything agrees with reason and is conducive to the good and benefit of one and all, then accept it and live up to it.

HINDU PRINCE GAUTAMA SIDDHARTA,
THE FOUNDER OF BUDDHISM, 563–483 B.C.

AFTERWORD

If you want to learn unconditional love, you must be prepared to confront all your conditions. In other words, to learn something, you must go through its opposite in order to attain it. To achieve a painless childbirth, you must experience pain—not necessarily physical pain, but the pain of change, of letting go of old habits, beliefs, resentments, behaviors, and attitudes. If we become conscious and act accordingly, not aspiring to be perfect human beings, but gathering the tools needed to reach a state of mental, physical, and spiritual well-being, we can change our experiences. If the only requirement for membership in the human race is to seek out love for oneself, love for one another, peace, joy, and appreciation for what we have, then we can make a difference. More and more, researchers are looking into the importance the parents' well-being during what Dr. Luzes[75] calls the fundamental five steps to a human being's life: conception, pregnancy, birth, breastfeeding, and the first three years of life. Cherishing and caring for every human being, beginning at conception or even before, could literally change the very biochemistry we have thought we were enslaved to. Dr. Luzes states, "If young people have a fundamental understanding of the five steps, they will have the ability to parent a new species: *Homo sapiens fraters* [brother.]"

The scientific community is waking up to the importance of imparting to young people a solution to our fast-paced and heartless living. When we nurture the new generation in our womb and teach them love for all the creatures of the universe, and as we show them how it is done through our example, we have a chance to survive global warming, to possibly eradicate world hunger, and to end war-mongering.

Oneness with all is only limited by a sense of separation that can be un-learned. The Nine Basic Human Rights are already yours; they are part of your inheritance, and inheritance is not earned, it is a birthright. But you cannot change the illusion of separateness unless you realize that the illusion is there. That's when the spiritual journey begins. Once we take ownership of our Nine Basic Human Rights, we transfer our renewed self-confidence directly into the very fiber that makes up our child's body, mind, and soul. I encourage you to seek other women on this journey. Together we can make a difference, and together we can bring back our right to have a painless, conscious, and sacred birthing experience.

APPENDIX:
CONVERSATIONS AT THE HOSPITAL

Even though I am a strong advocate for home birth, for I believe it is not only safe for both mom and child, but it is also the best environment, I also respect all those who choose a hospital birth. In 2006 I wrote an article entitled "Homebirth at the Hospital," which was published on *Mothering* magazine's Web site, www.mothering.com. As soon as it was online, I received a furious letter from someone who thought that I was selling "false hope" by even hinting at the possibility that a hospital birth could be at all similar to a homebirth. Yet more than 90 percent of all births in the United States are done in hospitals, and women deserve to be supported to achieve the most optimal experience no matter where they birth. Here is a quick checklist for you to read before you go to the hospital.

REMINDERS BEFORE YOU GO TO THE HOSPITAL

If you have planned a hospital birth or have to be transported to it after your homebirth did not go as planned, know that you now own all your basic human rights, your guardian angels are with you, and you have nature's power at hand. You are one with the universe and you are experiencing that which you were placed in this world to do.

There are two major reactions to entering the hospital—a conscious, rational one and an unconscious, emotional one.

Consciously, you have prepared yourself for this; you know you are simply using their facility, so you will bring "your home" with you, and you will continue to labor naturally with the help of your team. You'll abide by the rules that speak of their need to monitor the child's heartbeat for the first twenty minutes or half an hour, and their need to check you both vaginally and otherwise (blood pressure, temperature etc.) However, after you are admitted, you will move around, walk, and even take a shower if you need to cope with your contractions.

Unconsciously, your memories and knowledge of hospitals may still push you to think: "Hey, we are going to the hospital; something is wrong!" Further, most hospitals will insist that you sit in a wheelchair on your way to admission, once again making you feel powerless to even walk to your room, as if there is something seriously wrong with you. Stripped of your comfy, home clothes and asked to put on a hospital gown, you see yourself visually just like all other patients there, so you assume there must be something wrong with you. At this point, you will have to reason with your unconscious mind and keep reassuring the little child-self that all is well. Stop for a moment and write down an affirmation you can use in this moment that will remind you of what you are at the hospital to do and give you the confidence you need to consciously give birth. For example: "I am one with nature, all is well," or "All is well; I let go and let God."

Once at the hospital, the word game begins. Depending on the nursing staff and your care provider, once you enter into their territory, they will begin telling you what you should do, how you should do it, when and why you should or shouldn't, and how this is all for your own good. I have often heard phrases like: "You don't need to be a hero and take the pain; the health of the baby is the most important thing." Let me tell you, this is where all the work you have done so far really needs to come out if you want to have the kind of birthing experience you have been working toward, dreaming of, and are entitled to have.

First, I suggest that before you go to the hospital, you review your plan with your doula and support system. There is never truly a rush to go to the hospital unless it's an emergency, and if it's an emergency, then remember you are indeed a patient and, as such, armed with your information, you will then need to follow a different procedure. Assuming there is no emergency, review your Birth Plan. It will take only five minutes, and those few minutes can make a world of difference.

Remind yourself of the following: "I feel strong enough to walk to the maternity ward on my own two feet, and this will help my baby come down even more."

This can be the very first breakdown point; once they have convinced you that you must sit in the wheelchair, they have won their first battle.[76]

Be polite, but let the nurse know right away that *you* will be making all the decisions. When she asks for anything and you are about to manage a wave, tell her, "Just a moment, let me do this contraction and I'll answer your question." If you are beyond all these words, say "contraction" or raise a hand and go into your contraction meditation and she'll know you're not ready to talk. Make sure your team takes care of you and doesn't answer the questions for you (again, only if this is not an emergency). I am going to sound like a broken record about this, but this is an important point. We must make plans, but ultimately allow our reason and the situation to lead us.

As you are getting monitored, you might want to send your partner to talk to the head nurse to request a nurse who is supportive of natural childbirth, or you can ask the head nurse yourself. A word about nurses: nurses are not the enemy. Whatever they say to you, their intentions are good. They do and say what they have been used to doing and saying. They may have had a long day and dealing with a natural birth is a lot more work for them. They are caught between you and your doctor, and they want to please the doctor because they will work with him/her for many years to come and will see you only once or twice (if it is a small town) in their entire career. We need to make friends with our nurses. I suggest you mention your desire for a nurse who is supportive of natural childbirth on your Birth Plan and deliver it as soon as possible upon arriving into labor and delivery. Use the "head nurse method" only if you feel uncomfortable with the nurse that has welcomed you into the hospital.

After the baby's heartbeat and your contractions have been

monitored (and if all is well), they will want to check your cervix. Depending on the hospital, you will be checked either by the admitting nurse, an admitting midwife or, in case of a teaching hospital,[77] you will be checked by the resident. It is very unlikely at this point that your doctor will be at the hospital; however, if she is there, you will be checked by her. A word about residents: For the most part, residents are not students who do not know what they are doing. They have been through training and are supervised by a more experienced resident. That being said, I have had both amazing experiences and terrible ones with residents. Some, too green, inappropriately commented on what should be done, or erroneously measured the levels of waters, used a speculum for a vaginal exam, etc. In their favor, I have noticed that some have heard the latest research done on birth and the pros and cons of interventions. Thus, they might be even more inclined to natural childbirth than your doctor. Use your intuition and get in touch with the feeling you get once a young resident presents herself in front of you for a vaginal. It is your body. You choose who touches it!

At this point, there are several possible scenarios:

- Your waters are intact and you are less than five centimeters dilated. You could go home, take a vigorous walk, or take a bath. The best thing to do is to get out of the hospital and MOVE!

- Your waters have broken, but you are less than five centimeters. Be aware: most hospitals do not like you to go home once your waters are broken. However, if your baby is OK and if you feel like you can do it, sign your release and go home. If you stay, be prepared to hear talk of induction. You can choose what to do, but be cautious. Many times I have heard comments as mild as, "If you don't get induced, you might risk an infection," and as strong as, "If you don't get induced, your baby might die." Yes, unfortunately I have heard the last comment, which of course makes you feel like you're doing something to jeopardize the very life you're bringing into this world. It is true that once your waters break, there are risks of infections, but the percentages are fairly low. As long as you are willing to come back to be checked after twenty-four hours from the point the waters break, you should be OK. Most doctors are not comfortable with this scenario. I have heard several doctors and midwives confirm that it is perfectly safe for a woman to wait longer than twenty-four hours after her water breaks, but I suggest you discuss this with your care provider and choose your battles wisely. The best thing to do is to discuss this with your doctor ahead of time. Most physicians like to have the baby out no later than twenty-four hours after the amniotic sack ruptures; homebirth midwives have different rules. So if your water has recently broken, your baby is doing well, you do not have a fever, and overall you feel fine, there is no reason for you to stay at the hospital.

- Finally, you are five centimeters or more, and you can be admitted and checked into the delivery room even if your water has not broken. Settle down and continue with the management. If all is well, you do not need an IV fluid or to be monitored continuously. You can gently ask and agree to be monitored each hour for about twenty minutes (a good compromise with the nurse since it is her job on the line), but you will need to move around, change positions, and even take a walk in the corridors to keep things moving. If there is a shower or bathtub, ask to use it. It's great to settle into the hospital room after a relaxing, warm shower. Also, you might want to consider bringing a comfy nightgown with you. Make sure it's one that allows you to access your breasts easily (open in the front or spaghetti straps,) and short enough to get it out of the way for the birthing stage. You can probably use warm socks and slippers. If your waters have broken, you don't need to be checked often, as this will increase the chances of infection.

Now, let's talk about vaginal exams during your time in the hospital. Of course you'll need the initial one for evaluation and to decide whether you are going to be admitted or you are going to go back home. But once that's done, subsequent exams can work against you. In spite of the many things you'll hear such as, "You must dilate one centimeter per hour or you'll need to have a little Pitocin," each of our bodies reacts differently. You might get discouraged if you are checked too often. It's best to set a checking schedule you feel comfortable with (let's say every four to five hours) to simply monitor your progression. There is no rush in delivering babies as long as their heartbeat is steady between 120 and 180 BPM. A baby's heartbeat should not stay at the same number; a healthy birthing and laboring baby experiences many variations of heartbeat.

Hospital scenarios

- Once you get checked, here's what you may hear: "You've been laboring for quite some time and your cervix is still at 'X' centimeters dilated. I'd like you to consider Pitocin to kick start your labor and get this baby out." First of all, if they haven't suggested natural ways to induce your labor, ask to be given more time to try to progress naturally. Also, there are some natural ways the nurse or doctor can help the labor progress (like breaking the waters, helping you to move around, or suggesting you use a birthing ball). If the baby is not in trouble and her fetal heart patterns are normal, you should gently decline and ask them to give you more time to kick your labor into gear. Consider that the time of day and the day of the week might be a factor in this rash decision. Sometimes (not all the time), your provider wants to manage his/her schedule and time the birth to their convenience. Again, this is not done maliciously since (unfortunately) many doctors believe there is nothing wrong with inducing a patient. Yet research shows that the more medical interventions there are, the more likely the birth will turn into a Cesarean because either you or the baby will not respond well to the Pitocin. It's best to say something like, "I'm doing just fine, and if the baby is doing well I don't mind waiting for the natural course of things."

- After a few hours at the hospital, and after a check, you might hear the following: "You've been laboring for a while and we don't see any relative progression. This baby might be too big to fit through your pelvis; you should consider a Cesarean." Again, you must ask the right questions and consider all the factors involved. To avoid this, early on in your care and after an ultrasound, ask your provider if he/she thinks that your pelvis is big enough for the passage of your baby. Continue to ask this until the very last ultrasound. You can then use their words of reassurance and reiterate that if the baby's heartbeat is fine you would like to wait. Talk to the nurse (without the doctor) and to your doula and hear their opinions. Make sure you don't spend too much time in bed because the supine position will hinder the natural gravity pull of the baby.
- I have also heard this one: "You know, if you get an epidural, you will relax enough for your cervix to dilate." It's true, and I've seen this happen, yet it's important to realize that what they are saying is that you are tensing up at each contraction so much so that your uterus is working twice as hard. Tell them that you will try to work on relaxing more and would like to reevaluate the suggestion in a few hours. This is the time to work on your last fears and embrace the labor dance, determined to relax with each wave. It is not that I am 100 percent against epidurals. An epidural will indeed relax you, yet if it is done too early, it will stop or slow down your contractions, leading you to need Pitocin to re-start the contractions, and once again beginning the medical intervention spiral I mentioned in the pages on epidurals.
- You may hear: "Your baby is in distress, we need to perform a Cesarean." This is serious business and it is not said lightly. Nevertheless, if that is the case, you will have been alerted to the fact that the baby has been in distress (shown as an irregular or very slow heartbeat). For usually when that happens, the head nurse comes to your room and talks to your nurse about what has been happening. Often in the last stages, the

baby moves around and the umbilical cord gets pinched somewhere, thus decelerating his heartbeat. The best thing to do in such an occasion is to move around and even get up to see if the baby will move slightly to stabilize her own heartbeat. If you have an epidural, you often cannot move and certainly cannot stand up. Also, sometimes deceleration comes with high dosages of Pitocin, so just setting your Pitocin at a lower level or shutting it off completely can get the heartbeat steady. Make sure all those things are done before you even consider a Cesarean. Make sure the deceleration is not an isolated incidence, but that there has been a pattern in the last twenty minutes and that a shift in position has done nothing to change it. Again, talk to your nurse and doula in private and ask their opinion. They will be freer to talk to you without the doctor around. At times, doctors make those kinds of statements and will not leave the room. I found that a great way to have some privacy is to say, "OK, I'd like to pray right now." And you'll see doctors run out of the room as fast as the speed of light! If this is a true emergency, it may seem that there is no time to take a private moment. At that point, you must let go and prepare yourself for a different kind of birth. Even if only for a few moments, do pray or meditate and share this space with your team to center before you change gears.

- You may hear: "If you are not at 'x' centimeters when I call next time, I'd like to start Pitocin." This sounds unreasonable since we cannot put the baby and labor on a schedule. Again, if the baby is doing OK, ask to be left alone and let your body progress at its own pace. I once had a doctor get so mad when a client said this, that she demanded to speak with me. I declined, telling her that the decision was my client's, not mine, and that she should talk to her directly. Remember, the relationship and all decisions are up to you, not your partner or your doula. Definitely ask for their support and counsel, but stand up for yourself. Show your child you are in charge and that it is safe to come, for you are capable of taking care of her.

- You may hear: "You have been pushing for a while and the baby is not coming out. We need to do a C-section." Every doctor and hospital has set times they will allow you to push before they perform a Cesarean. In reality, there are no real set times. I had a client push as long as five hours. If the baby's heartbeat is fine, there is no hurry to get the baby out. Once presented with such a statement, angelically ask, "Is the baby's heartbeat OK? Can I hear it? Is he in distress?" If the answer is no, then ask for more time. Stand up and use gravity to help you. One squat is worth twenty supine pushes. Close your eyes and talk to your baby. Make sure to tell him you are ready to embrace him and that this would be a good time to come out. You can squat in bed with an epidural with the help of your team.

- You may hear: "I need to do an episiotomy to get this baby out." More often than not, doctors who do an episiotomy as a routine will not even ask you or tell you they are going to do it. It is important that you have discussed your desires with them beforehand and that your partner is ready to keep an eye out for you (you might not be in a position to see what's going on). If your partner sees the doctor taking the scissors, make sure he/she asks why the provider thinks you need an episiotomy. One thing I often do as a doula is praise my client out loud during the pushing stages with phrases like: "Wow, your perineum is really stretching well, I don't think you're even going to tear," or "The baby's heartbeat is so nice and healthy, aren't you lucky you don't seem to need an episiotomy!" I have seen doctors pick up the scissors a couple of times and then put them down after such comments. I also encourage you to touch your baby's head as soon as it peeks through the vaginal opening. The more your hands wander down there, the less likely your doctor will be to give you an episiotomy.

Find your own voice, be your own advocate, participate in your care and decision making. You will feel much more confident as a person and later as a mother, and no matter the outcome, you will not feel like a victim. In the final analysis, doctors will welcome this, for the responsibility of all the choices will not rest on their shoulders alone and fewer malpractice suits will ensue.

HOMEBIRTH AT THE HOSPITAL

No matter where you are going to give birth to your child, focus on the birthing, the sacredness of the experience, and your co-participation with your child in the miracle at hand, no matter the circumstances.

There are five steps to help you realize your desire for a home-like, natural, and painless childbirth at the hospital:

1. *Be willing to have a natural experience, no matter what.* Be willing to change what you believe and what you have been taught. In order to change our intention and the outcome of any of our endeavors, we need to start by becoming clear as to what we want. Have a clear intention of the kind of birthing experience you want, regardless of what you have heard, what kind of birth your mother, sisters, etc. had, and regardless of your age, size, heritage, and so forth. The fact that you are reading this book is already a wonderful step in that direction. Consider hiring a doula, taking an independent childbirth education class, and talking to women who have experienced natural childbirth.

2. *Trust that you can do it.* Believing not only that you can do it but that you deserve to have such an experience is a very important step toward success. Tell yourself every day that you will have the birthing experience you desire. Write it down, meditate on it, and pray for it. Do whatever it takes to grow the self-confidence that you have all it takes to have such an experience. Make sure you surround yourself with supportive people. Do not waste time listening to those who are quick to tell you that

it is impossible, or those who would like you to have the same medicated experience they had.

3. *Make the decision that a natural childbirth and homelike birth experience is what you want and will have.* The first two steps had to do with an inner dialogue. This step suggests that you no longer vacillate about your intention. If you have chosen to have your child at the hospital because you feel more comfortable, you have made a good decision, because you based your decision on how you feel and what you desire. Now, decide that you will have a homelike birth at the hospital of your choice. Make sure you choose a hospital that will allow you to have such an experience. Go and visit the hospitals that are covered by your insurance company. Ask other women, doulas, childcare educators, and midwives about each facility, so you can make a truly informed decision.

4. *Take action.* Choose a care provider that will support your desire. Interview a few; make sure they have supported other women who had the same experience you want. Ask the doctors if they are willing to give you the names of patients who have had a natural childbirth, so that you may talk to them and get some advice. Be diligent and empowered; ask as many questions as you can think of, and then ask more. Go to independent childbirth education classes, look into hypnosis for a painless childbirth, hire a doula (visit DONA.org to find a certified doula in your area,) and find alternative ways to cope with labor.

5. *Share your joyful experience with others.* Because you have been successful obtaining a natural, homelike birth at the hospital, share your experience with other women and help them fulfill their desires and dreams. If you can do it, we can all do it. Share the joy.

NOTES

1. "A Birth Doula is a woman experienced in childbirth who provides continuous physical, emotional, and informational support to the mother before, during, and just after childbirth." Marshall H. Klaus, John H. Kennell, and Phyllis H. Klaus, *Mothering the Mother: How a Doula Can Help You Have a Shorter, Easier, and Healthier Birth* (Addison Wesley, 1993).

2. Neonatologist Jean-Pierre Relier's research on very early cellular distribution of IGF (intrauterine growth hormone).

3. "Early Childhood Influences on a Woman's Later Childbearing," presentation by Penny Simkin at the 12th annual International Dona's conference in Denver Colorado.

4. Penny Simkin and Phyllis Klaus, *When Survivors Give Birth: Understanding and Healing the Effects of Early Sexual Abuse on Childbearing Women* (Seattle, Wash.: Classic Day, 2004).

5. When the back of the baby's head faces toward the mother's back, creating added pressure in the laboring woman.

6. I joined Co-Dependents Anonymous. For more information and for their literature please visit www.coda.org.

7. *Big Book of Alcoholics Anonymous.*

8. A version is a manual manipulation performed by a doctor in the attempt to turn a breech baby. Often, versions are done by the thirty-eighth week of gestation, usually under anesthesia. As most breech babies nowadays are delivered by Cesarean, doctors usually don't perform versions during labor

9. Elizabeth M. Carman and Neil J. Carman, *Cosmic Cradle: Souls Waiting in the Wings for Birth* (Fairfield, Iowa: Sunstar Pub., 1999).

10. Carolyn Myss, *Sacred Contracts: Awakening Your Divine Potential* (New York: Harmony Books, 2001).

11. Wayne Muller, *How Then, Shall We Live? Four Simple Questions That Reveal the Beauty and Meaning of Our Lives* (New York: Bantam, 1996).

12. Ina May Gaskin, *Spiritual Midwifery,* 4th ed. (Summerville, Tenn.: Book Publishing Company, 2002).

13. Rudolf Steiner, Clopper Almon, and Catherine E. Creeger, *An Outline of Esoteric Science* (SteinerBooks, Foundational Work).

14. David Chamberlain, Ed., *Early Parenting Is Prenatal Parenting!* www.birthpsychology.com.

15. Ibid.

16. Some of these questions have been adapted from the Mother Friendly Childbirth Initiative; visit them at www.motherfriendly.org.

17. Kangaroo care happens when the mother of a preemie is allowed to hold the baby next to her skin in a kangaroo-style wrapping. To learn more visit www.kangaroomothercare.com.

18. Chapter seven has a lot of suggestions regarding breech babies and what you can do in case your baby is not head first.

19. "Home Births Safe for Most," article published on Feb. 6, 2002, by Web MD, citing a study published in the *Canadian Medical Association Journal*, www.webmd.com.

20. M. J. Lafuente, R. Grifol, J. Segarra, J. Soriano, M.A. Gorba, and A. Montesinos, "Effects of the Firstart Method of Prenatal Stimulation on Psychomotor Development: The First Six Months," *Journal of Prenatal & Perinatal Psychology & Health*, 11, no. 3 (1997): 151–162.

21. Ibid.

22. Amniocentesis is a prenatal test that allows your healthcare practitioner to gather information about your baby's health and development from a sample of your amniotic fluid.

23. Marshall H. Klaus, John H. Kennell, and Phyllis H. Klaus, *Mothering the Mother: How a Doula Can Help You Have a Shorter, Easier, and Healthier Birth* (Reading, Mass.: Addison-Wesley, 1993).

24. *A Course in Miracles*, publication of the Foundation for Inner Peace.

25. This guided meditation is also available on my Web site at www.joyinbirthing.com.

26. A cheesy, white substance that covers a baby's skin at birth. Without the vernix, the baby would have very wrinkled skin from constant exposure to the watery amniotic fluid.

27. Written on December 10, 1948, by the General Assembly of the United Nations.

28. Bruce Lipton, Ph.D., "The Wisdom of your Cells," www.brucelipton.com.

29. Serenity prayer, Alcoholics Anonymous.

30. Nesting is the term used when a mother or a couple feel an uncontrollable urge to clean their house. It is brought on by a desire to prepare a nest for the new baby, to tie up loose ends of old projects, and to organize your world.

31. Found on the Life Before Birth Web site, www.birthpsychology.com.

32. Bruce Lipton, Ph.D., "The Wisdom of your Cells," www.brucelipton.com.

33. *Journal of Pediatrics*, August 2007 edition, conducted by Frederick J. Zimmerman, Dimitri A. Christakis, and Andrew Metzoff.

34. A heplock is an IV site (a small catheter inserted in a vein usually on the wrist or the hand) ready in case you need to be given medication or fluids. It's freestanding and does not need to be hooked up to any IV fluids.

35. One minute and then five minutes after the birth, a score is given rating the baby's activity (muscle tone), pulse, grimace (reflex irritability), appearance (skin color), and respiration. If there are problems with the baby, an additional score is given at ten minutes. A score of 7–10 is considered normal, while 4–7 might require some resuscitative measures, and a baby with Apgars of 3 and below requires immediate resuscitation.

36. E-book available on line at www.joyinbirthing.com.

37. Carl Jones, *Mind over Labor* (New York: Penguin, 1988, 1987).

38. Downy hair on the body of the fetus and newborn baby.

39. John E. Upledger, D.O., O.M.M., *A Brain Is Born: Exploring the Birth and Development of the Central Nervous System* (Berkeley, Calif.: North Atlantic Books, 1996).

40. I do not recommend you do this alone if the memory is violent or if it truly has been a traumatic event. It is best is to enlist a professional to help you on your journey.

41. The "babymoon" is what Katzinger calls the period immediately following the baby's birth, when we go on a honeymoon with our child and our partner.

42. This can sound scary, especially since it's very common to vomit during active labor or transition. Please know that this information is provided to make you aware of how important it is to keep your body fueled for the work ahead. Other research has indicated that severe restriction on oral intake (as in no food at all during a woman's hospital stay while in labor) can lead to ketosis.

43. Thrush is an infection of the mouth caused by the *Candida* fungus. Visit www.drjaygordon.com to get great information on breastfeeding and how to cope with thrush.

44. Thorp J. A., and Breedlove, G., "Epidural Analgesia in Labor: An Evaluation of the Risks and Benefits," *Birth* 23:2 (1996).

45. Walker, M., "Do Labor Medications Affect Breastfeeding?" *Journal of Human Lactation* 13, no. 2, (1997): 131–7.

46. Although I strongly believe in positive thinking, I'm also a proponent of gaining knowledge in all aspects of birthing. Important decisions such as what to do if the baby needs to go to NICU (neonatal intensive care unit) or in case of a Cesarean birth should be the result of informed consent.

47. Braxton Hicks contractions are sporadic uterine contractions that actually start very early in pregnancy, but most women don't feel them until the last trimester.

48. David B. Chamberlain, Ph.D., *The Fetal Senses: A Classical View*, (Birnholz, 1981), www.birthpsychology.com.

49. Toffelmier, Gertrude, and Luomala, Katherine, "Dreams and Dream Interpretation of the Diegueno Indians of Southern California," *The Psychoanalytic Quarterly* 5 (1936): 195–225

50. A derogative word used to label a person from the South, literally translating as "of the earth" or "made of dirt."

51. "Giuditta speaks through her nose."

52. "What's the matter, darling?"

53. Sheila Kitzinger. *Rediscovering Birth* (New York: Pocket Books, 2000).

54. Ibid.

55. This is called spinning the baby. Visit www.spinningbabies.com for more information on this technique.

56. John E. Upledger, D.O., O.M.M., *A Brain Is Born: Exploring the Birth and Development of the Central Nervous System* (Berkeley, Cal.: North Atlantic Books, 1996).

57. Italo Calvino, *t zero* (New York : Harcourt Brace Jovanovich, 1976, 1969).

58. C. L. Paseo and R. Britt, "Managing Pain During Labor," *American Journal of Nursing* 98 (August 1998: 10–11).

59. Nancy Lowe "The Name of Labor Pain," *American Journal of Obstetrics and Gynecology* 186, no. 5 (May 2002, Suppl: S16-S24).

60. E. R. Cluett, V. C. Nikodem, R. E. McCandlish, and E. E. Burs, "Immersion in Water in Pregnancy, Labor and Birth," *The Cochrane Database of Systematic Reviews* 2 (2004: CD000111).

61. A. Cyna, G. McAuliffe, and M. Andrew, "Hypnosis for Pain Relief in Labor and Childbirth: A Systematic Review," *British Journal of Anesthesia* 93, no. 4 (2004: 505–11).

62. Bloom et al., "A Randomized Trial of Coached Versus Uncoached Maternal Pushing During the Second Stage of Labor," *American Journal of Obstetrics and Gynecology* (January 2006).

63. *Laboring Down:* Allowing your body to push the baby out on its own.

64. Bloom et al., "A Randomized Trial of Coached Versus Uncoached Maternal Pushing During the Second Stage of Labor," *American Journal of Obstetrics and Gynecology* (January 2006).

65. The most common position for a baby during labor is head-down with the back of the head (occiput) facing the front of the mother (anterior). OP refers to *occiput posterior,* that is when the back of the baby's head faces the back and you are likely to experience back labor. OT refers to *occiput transverse,* that's when the baby's head faces the side.

66. Sarah Buckley, MD, "Leaving Well Alone: A Natural Approach to the Third Stage of Labour," www.childbirthsolutions.com.

67. Sermon—Dr. Michael Beckweth, Agape International Spiritual Center, Culver City, California.

68. Instead of just treating specific symptoms, osteopathic physicians concentrate on treating you as a whole. They focus special attention on the musculoskeletal system, which reflects and influences the condition of all other body systems.

69. Written by Magaret Sorrel, D.O., F.C.A., for the Cranial Academy.

70. A table used to determine how successful an induction of labor might be. It is recommended that the Bishop's Score be greater than 9 for induction to be successful.

71. The Webster Technique, discovered by Dr. Larry Webster, founder of the International Chiropractic Pediatric Association (ICPA), is a specific chiropractic adjustment for pregnant mothers. It is a chiropractic technique designed to relieve the causes of intrauterine constraint.

72. For more information, contact the Postpartum Stress Center, (610) 525–7527; Postpartum Support International, (800) 944–4773; or the National Institute

of Mental Health, (800) 421–4211. Also visit http://www.postpartum.net/ http://www.depressionafterdelivery.com/

73. Klaus, M., Fox, N., & Keefe, M. R. (1998). *The Amazing Talents of the Newborn* (video). Johnson & Johnson. To purchase this video call 1-877-565-5465.

74. T Berry Brazelton, M.D., Joshua D. Sparrow, *Sleep : The Brazelton Way* (Cambridge, Mass.: Perseus, 2003).

75. Dr. Eleanor Madruga Lunez, MD, psychiatrist and Jungian analyst from Rio de Janeiro, Brazil.

76. Please, I expect you to use common sense. If you can't walk, then don't! I have had clients who have gotten to the hospital in transition and needed to sit. Do so as long as it is *your* decision and not an "abdication" on your part.

77. A teaching hospital is one where graduate students of medicine do their internships before finishing their medical degree and going on their own practice.

ABOUT THE AUTHOR

Giuditta Tornetta experienced her own painless childbirth in 1984, and the experience inspired her to dedicate her life to helping women obtain painless, natural childbirth. A birth and postpartum doula, she is also a lactation educator, a clinical hypnotherapist, and an NLP (neuro-linguistic programming) practitioner. A contributing editor for *Los Angeles Family* magazine with her monthly column, "Ask Doula Giuditta," *Las Vegas Family* magazine, *The Wet Set Gazette,* and SheKnows.com, Tornetta has published more than 300 articles in the United States and United Kingdom. Excerpts from this book have appeared in *The Mother* magazine in the United Kingdom and *Mothering* magazine in the United States.